International Ophthalmology Clinics

International Ophthalmology Clinics (ISSN 0020-8167) (ISBN 0-316-29417-9). Published quarterly by Little, Brown and Company, 34 Beacon Street, Boston, Massachusetts 02108-1493. Send address changes and subscription orders to Little, Brown and Company, Subscription Department, 34 Beacon St, Boston, MA 02108. Subscription rates per year: personal subscription, U.S. and possessions, $99; foreign (includes Mexico), $129; Canada, $115, PLEASE ADD 7% CANADIAN GST FOR ALL CANADIAN SUBSCRIPTIONS (Registration No. R128537917); institutional, U.S., $125; foreign, $165; Canada, $140. Special rates for students, interns and residents per year: U.S., $69; foreign, $95; Canada, $79. Single copies: $31 for subscribers, $39 for nonsubscribers. In Japan please contact our exclusive agent: Medsi, 1-2-13 Yushima, Bunkyo-ku, Tokyo 113, Japan. Subscription rates per year in Japan: individual, ¥25,800; institutional, ¥31,400 (air cargo service only). Second-class postage paid at Boston, Massachusetts, and at additional mailing offices.

Postmaster: Send address changes to International Ophthalmology Clinics, 34 Beacon St, Boston, MA 02108.

Copyright © 1994 by Little, Brown and Company (Inc). All rights reserved. Except as authorized in the accompanying statement no part of this publication may be reproduced in any form or by any electronic or mechanical means, including information storage and retrieval systems, without permission in writing from the publisher, except by a reviewer who may quote brief passages in a review to be printed in a magazine or newspaper.

Authorization to photocopy items for internal or personal use, or the internal or personal use of specific clients, is granted by Little, Brown and Company (Inc) for libraries and other users registered with the Copyright Clearance Center Transactional Reporting Service, provided that the per-copy fee of $3.00 is paid directly to the Copyright Clearance Center, 27 Congress St., Salem, MA 01970, for copying beyond that permitted by Sections 107 or 108 of the U.S. Copyright Law. The code fee for this journal is 0020-8167/94 $3.00. This authorization does not extend to other kinds of copying, such as copying for general distribution, for advertising or promotional purposes, for creating new collective works, or for resale. Copying fees for material published in this journal prior to January 1, 1978, will be charged according to fee rates on file with the Copyright Clearance Center, Inc.

International Ophthalmology Clinics is indexed in Index Medicus, Current Contents/Clinical Medicine, Excerpta Medica, and Current Awareness in Biological Sciences.

International Ophthalmology Clinics

Volume 34
Number 1
Winter 1994

Dry Eye

Little, Brown and Company
BOSTON

Editors

Gilbert Smolin, M.D.
F.I. Proctor Foundation, San Francisco
Department of Ophthalmology,
University of California, San Francisco
Medical Center

Mitchell H. Friedlaender, M.D.
Division of Ophthalmology,
Scripps Clinic and Research Foundation,
La Jolla, California

Editorial Office
1001 Sneath Lane, Room 206
San Bruno, CA 94066

Publisher
Little, Brown and Company, Boston, Massachusetts

Publishing Staff

Publisher
Thomas A. Manning

Executive Editor
David Dionne

Managing Editor
Maureen A. Hurley

Sales and Marketing Manager
Anne Orens

Production Manager
Fredda Purgalin

Editorial Board

Rubens Belfort, Jr., M.D., Sao Paulo, Brazil

David BenEzra, M.D., Jerusalem, Israel

Etienne Bloch Michel, M.D., Paris, France

Roger Buckley, F.R.C.S., London, England

Gunther Grabner, M.D., Vienna, Austria

Creig Hoyt, M.D., San Francisco, California

Bruce Jackson, M.D., Ottawa, Canada

Frederick Jakobiec, M.D., Boston, Massachusetts

Hector Maclean, M.D., East Melbourne, Australia

Yuichi Ohashi, M.D., Ehime, Japan

Shigeaki Ohno, M.D., Yokahama, Japan

Yves Pouliquen, M.D., Paris, France

Manuel Quintana, M.D., Barcelona, Spain

Rainer Sundmacher, M.D., Dusseldorf, Germany

Khalid Tabbara, M.D., Riyadh, Saudi Arabia

Eberhart Zrenner, M.D., Tübingen, Germany

Contents

- **Contributing Authors** ix

- **Preface** xiii
  Mitchell H. Friedlaender, M.D.

- **Autoimmunity of the Lacrimal Gland** 1
  Austin K. Mircheff, Ph.D.,
  J. Peter Gierow, Ph.D., and
  Richard L. Wood, Ph.D.

- **Hormonal Influences on the Lacrimal Gland** 19
  Dwight W. Warren, Ph.D.

- **Human Tear Film Electrolyte Concentrations in Health and Dry-Eye Disease** 27
  Jeffrey P. Gilbard, M.D.

- **Diagnosis of Keratoconjunctivitis Sicca** 37
  J. Daniel Nelson, M.D., F.A.C.S.

- **Evaluation of the Ocular Surface in Dry-Eye Conditions** 57
  Scheffer C. G. Tseng, M.D., Ph.D.

- **Systemic Diseases Associated with Dry Eye** 71
  Robert I. Fox, M.D., Ph.D.

- **Oral Disease Associated with Dry Eyes** 89
  Regina H. M. Kurrasch, M.D.,
  Ava J. Wu, D.D.S., and Philip C. Fox, D.D.S.

- **Management of the Dry-Eye Patient** 101
  Michael A. Lemp, M.D.

- **New Approaches to Dry-Eye Therapy**   115
  Kazuo Tsubota, M.D.

- **Contact Lenses and the Dry Eye**   129
  R. Linsy Farris, M.D.

- **Possible Mechanisms of Cellular Activation and Tissue Destruction in Sjögren's Syndrome**   137
  Ichiro Saito, D.D.S., Ph.D.

- **Punctal Occlusion**   145
  David W. Lamberts, M.D.

- **Abstracts**   151

- *Index*   167

Contributing Authors

R. Linsy Farris, M.D.
College of Physicians and Surgeons
Columbia University
New York, NY 10032

Philip C. Fox, D.D.S.
National Institutes of Health
Building 10, Room 1N-113
Bethesda, MD 20892

Robert I. Fox, M.D., Ph.D.
Departments of Rheumatology and Immunology
Scripps Clinic and Research Foundation
10666 North Torrey Pines Road
La Jolla, CA 92037

J. Peter Gierow, Ph.D.
Department of Pharmacology and Nutrition
University of Southern California School of Medicine
1975 Zonal Avenue
Los Angeles, CA 90033

Jeffrey P. Gilbard, M.D.
Department of Ophthalmology
Harvard Medical School
Boston, MA
Address correspondence to:
7 Alfred Street, Suite 330
Woburn, MA 01801

Regina H. M. Kurrasch, M.D.
National Institutes of Health
Building 10, Room 1N-113
Bethesda, MD 20892

David W. Lamberts, M.D.
Department of Ophthalmology
University Medical Center
Address correspondence to:
4003 22nd Street
Lubbock, TX 79410

Michael A. Lemp, M.D.
Department of Ophthalmology
Georgetown University Medical School
Address correspondence to:
4910 Massachusetts Avenue, NW
Suite 210
Washington, DC 20016

Austin K. Mircheff, Ph.D.
Department of Physiology and Biophysics
University of Southern California School of Medicine
1333 San Pablo Street
Los Angeles, CA 90033

J. Daniel Nelson, M.D., F.A.C.S.
Department of Ophthalmology
University of Minnesota
Minneapolis, MN
Address correspondence to:
640 Jackson Street
St. Paul, MN 55101

Ichiro Saito, D.D.S., Ph.D.
Division of Immunological Diseases
Medical Research Institute
Tokyo Medical and Dental University
1-5-45, Yushima, Bunkyo-ku
Tokyo 113, Japan

Scheffer C. G. Tseng, M.D., Ph.D.
Department of Ophthalmology
Bascom Palmer Eye Institute
University of Miami
Address correspondence to:
P.O. Box 016880
Miami, FL 33101

Kazuo Tsubota, M.D.
Department of Ophthalmology
Keio University School of Medicine
Tokyo, Japan
Address correspondence to:
5-11-13 Sugano
Ichikawa, Chiba 272 Japan

Dwight W. Warren, Ph.D.
Pharmacology and Nutrition
University of Southern California
1975 Zonal Avenue
Los Angeles, CA 90033

Richard L. Wood, Ph.D.
Anatomy and Cell Biology
University of Southern California
1333 San Pablo Street, BMT 401
Los Angeles, CA 90033

Ava J. Wu, D.D.S.
National Institutes of Health
Building 10, Room 1N-113
Bethesda, MD 20892

Preface

During my residency training, the terms "dry eye" and Sjögren's syndrome were mentioned a great deal. In fact, it was probably one of the few programs where Sjögren's name was pronounced correctly, since our chief, Claes Dohlman, was of Swedish origin, and had even met Sjögren, also a Swedish ophthalmologist. I thought I knew a fair amount about dry eyes at the time, especially after taking a cornea fellowship and developing a research interest in ocular immunology. In subsequent years, I believe I have made two valid observations about the dry eye. First, a lot of patients are told they have dry eyes when, in reality, they have some other external ocular condition, usually blepharitis. Second, there are at least two forms of dry eye: a mild form which is common and associated with the aging process; and a severe form, almost always found in women who are middle-aged or older, and associated with a dry mouth or a collagen-vascular disease. It is this latter group which fits the classic Sjögren's syndrome category.

Much of my personal knowledge about the dry eye stems from experience during the last 7 years at Scripps Clinic and Research Foundation. There, under the direction of Dr Robert Fox, Sjögren's syndrome patients are carefully evaluated through clinical and laboratory studies. We also use a helpful "team" approach in which patients have appointments with a rheumatologist, ophthalmologist, oral medicine specialist, and when necessary, a gynecologist, allergist, otorhinolaryngologist, and even a dermatologist. This team approach serves at least two purposes: it provides the Sjögren's patient with expertise in treating each system affected by this multi-faceted disease, and it allows the doctors the opportunity to confirm their diagnoses and develop an overall plan that will be most beneficial to the patient. While this team approach is best suited to multi-specialty groups and universities, I would recommend it to anyone involved in the care of Sjögren's syndrome patients.

This issue of *International Ophthalmology Clinics* provides us with an opportunity to review and update many of the important developments in the field of dry-eye and autoimmune diseases. Dr Mircheff and Dr Warren have pioneered some fascinating developments on the influence of hormones and the immune system on the production of tears. Dr Saito has taken this opportunity to study the pathology of destructive changes in the lacrimal gland in Sjögren's syndrome; Dr Tseng has provided new insights into the nature of tear film and the ocular surface; Dr Gilbard's studies on tear chemistry have provided us with a rationale for the development of better artificial tears; Dr Tsubota has developed some innovative approaches to diagnosis and treatment of the dry eye. We have also included superb reviews of the systemic nature of the disease by Dr Robert Fox, the oral manifestations by Dr Philip Fox, and an extensive review of the ocular findings by Dr Lemp and Dr Nelson. Finally, we have some special considerations about dry eyes and contact lenses by Dr Farris, and an overview of punctal occlusion by Dr Lamberts.

I believe this will be one of the most comprehensive and useful monographs on the dry eye. Our patients with these distressing, but manageable, conditions will be the ultimate beneficiaries of this issue of *International Ophthalmology Clinics*.

Mitchell H. Friedlaender

Autoimmunity of the Lacrimal Gland

Austin K. Mircheff, Ph.D.
J. Peter Gierow, Ph.D.
Richard L. Wood, Ph.D.

■ Lacrimal Secretion

The lacrimal glands secrete a mixture of proteins, nutrients, hormones, growth factors, and immunoglobulins in an approximately isotonic electrolyte solution. Lacrimal acinar cells release secretory proteins, such as lysozyme and lactoferrin, by the classical merocrine mechanism. The acini use transcytotic mechanisms to secrete immunoglobulins, primarily secretory immunoglobulin A (IgA), and at least one protein hormone, prolactin [1, 2]. Lacrimal duct cells contain epidermal growth factor (EGF) [3], and they appear to release it both into the forming lacrimal gland fluid and into the lacrimal interstitium, where it may function as a paracrine mediator.

■ Chronic Inflammatory Processes

The lacrimal glands normally contain populations of plasma cells, which produce the dimeric IgA that is secreted into lacrimal gland fluid [4], smaller numbers of T lymphocytes, and even smaller numbers of B lymphocytes [5]. Within the population of T lymphocytes, suppressor cells normally outnumber helper cells by a two- to threefold margin [5, 6].

It is widely appreciated that in Sjögren's syndrome, the number of lymphocytes infiltrating the lacrimal glands increases markedly [7–9], whereas the secretory epithelial tissue atrophies, ultimately to be replaced by fibrous connective tissue. The loss of epithelial tissue certainly must account for the pronounced sicca symptoms in Sjögren's syndrome, but it also seems likely that factors released by the infiltrating lymphocytes interfere with epithelial function during the earlier progress of the disease. Analogous histopathological and functional changes frequently occur also in the salivary glands, with resulting xerostomia. The increased number of lymphocytes results primarily from expansion of the helper subset of T lymphocytes [9, 10] and the appearance of large numbers of IgG-secreting B lymphocytes. The expanded lymphocyte populations are distributed diffusely as well as concentrated in foci; occasionally, epimyoepithelial islands containing small numbers of dendritic cells in addition to the T and B lymphocytes are also present. More than one focus of 50 or more cells per 4 mm^2 of tissue frequently is a required criterion for diagnosis of Sjögren's syndrome. The hypergamaglobulinemia and circulating autoantibodies typical of Sjögren's syndrome are produced, at least in part, by lacrimal and salivary gland–resident B cells [11].

There are many uncertainties associated with diagnosis of lacrimal insufficiency, and adequate epidemiological statistics have not been collected. However, it is clear that sicca symptoms are widespread in the elderly population and that they afflict many individuals who do not exhibit the serological abnormalities characteristic of Sjögren's syndrome or other systemic immune disorders [12]. In a study of patients presenting with aqueous insufficiency at a dry-eye clinic, roughly 40% lacked either subjective or objective signs of xerostomia. This group also exhibited lower incidences of antinuclear antibodies, rheumatoid factor, and hypergamaglobulinemia, and they failed to exhibit antibodies to Ro(SS-A) and La(SS-B) [13]. In a population of elderly women, 24% had positive Schirmer's I tests (less than 6 mm of wetting in 5 minutes), whereas only 2% clearly satisfied the diagnosis of Sjögren's syndrome and an additional 12% were classified with possible Sjögren's syndrome [14]. In a study of patients presenting with sicca symptoms at a rheumatology clinic, the symptoms of patients for whom the diagnosis of Sjögren's syndrome could be excluded were indistinguishable from the symptoms of those for whom the diagnosis of Sjögren's syndrome could be confirmed [15].

Non-Sjögren's sicca symptoms are typically attributed to senile atrophy of the lacrimal gland. As Warren argues elsewhere (see the chapter, "Hormonal Influences on the Lacrimal Gland"), much of the age-related decrement in lacrimal secretory function appears to result from loss of hormonal support for the lacrimal secretory epithelium. However, it is likely that excessive lymphocytic proliferation is an additional compounding factor. In a study of lacrimal glands obtained at autopsy, lymphocytic focus scores of greater than one per 4 mm^2 were observed in 12% of the cases [16], although this appeared to be accompanied only rarely by acinar atrophy or fibrosis. In another postmortem study, lymphocytic infiltration of the lacrimal glands was observed to increase with age and to be accompanied by fibrosis and acinar atrophy, though the massive destruction of secretory epithelial tissue characteristic of Sjögren's syndrome was not observed [17].

Thus, it seems plausible to hypothesize that excessive proliferation of T lymphocytes, perhaps distributed in normal proportions between helper and suppressor subsets and unaccompanied by proliferation of B cells and consequent serological abnormalities, may contribute to sicca symptoms in a significant number of cases.

In the remainder of this chapter, we discuss mechanisms that may trigger and perpetuate the excessive accumulation of T and B lymphocytes. Two different theories merit close attention. One focuses on the role viral infections may play, the other on the role played by epithelial cells aberrantly expressing class II histocompatibility molecules.

■ Role of Viral Infections

A number of investigators have explored the possibility that viral infections may initiate autoimmune phenomena, either by altering antigen presentation or by influencing fundamental aspects of the immune response [18]. The herpesviruses have attracted the most attention. One early suggestion was that persistent cytomegalovirus (CMV) infection played a role in the etiology of Sjögren's syndrome [19]. More recently, attention has turned to Epstein-Barr virus (EBV): Several groups have reported development of Sjögren's syndrome in patients with infectious mononucleosis [20, 21]. Fox and coworkers [22] detected EBV antigens in salivary glands but not in other tissues from 8 of 14 Sjögren's syndrome patients. Mariette and colleagues [23] detected EBV genes in salivary glands from 6 of 7 primary Sjögren's patients, 3 of 5 secondary Sjögren's patients, and 7 of 24 control subjects. Similarly, using the polymerase chain reaction, Pflugfelder and associates [24] detected EBV genes in 8 of 10 lacrimal glands from Sjögren's patients who were seropositive for EBV antigens. This same group was able to detect EBV antigens in 2 of 6 Sjögren's lacrimal glands but in none of the controls examined [25], and they noted a correlation between levels of serum antibodies to EBV antigens and the severity of aqueous tear deficiency. There remains some controversy about the significance of such observations, however. EBV genomic sequences frequently are found in normal lacrimal tissues [26], and Deacon and coworkers [27] contend that EBV DNA can be detected with equal frequencies in normal salivary glands and in salivary glands from primary and secondary Sjögren's syndrome patients. Fox and Kang [28] have raised the possibility that reactivation of EBV is a consequence, rather than a cause, of immunoproliferation in the salivary and lacrimal glands in Sjögren's syndrome. Nonetheless, several specific mechanisms by which EBV participates in the immunopathogenesis of Sjögren's syndrome can be envisioned.

Some evidence has been presented suggesting a role of retroviruses in the development of Sjögren's and Sjögren's-like lymphoproliferation in the exocrine glands. Garry and coworkers [29] have detected retroviral particles antigenically similar to the human immunodeficiency virus (HIV) in extracts of salivary glands from 2 of 6 Sjögren's patients. Keratoconjunctivitis sicca, confirmed with both Schirmer's and tear osmolarity tests, has been noted in 21% of a sample of acquired immunodeficiency syndrome (AIDS) patients [30]. In a sample of AIDS patients with xerostomia who were tested, all exhibited lymphocytic focus scores of two or more. Notably, however, the predominant T-cell population was of the suppressor (CD8) subset, in contrast to the helper subset characteristic of Sjögren's syndrome [31].

Several hypotheses have been suggested to account for the mechanisms by which viruses influence Sjögren's and Sjögren's-like lymphocytic proliferation. One is molecular mimicry, whereby viral proteins that provoke immune responses mimic normal cellular proteins. For example, Talal and colleagues [32] have noted that the p24 gag protein of HIV-1 shares an epitope with a nucleoprotein (Sm) against which antibodies are made in some systemic lupus erythematosus and Sjögren's patients. It has also been suggested that infecting viruses program cellular production of autocrine growth factors [33, 34]. One particular attraction of this hypothesis is that autocrine growth stimulation, perhaps accompanied by antigen-driven T-lymphocyte activation, could reasonably account for the oligoclonal character of the B cell infiltrates observed in many Sjögren's patients and for the 40-fold greater tendency of B-cell malignancies to arise in Sjögren's patients.

■ Role of Aberrant Class II Histocompatibility Antigen Expression

After observing that thyroid epithelial cells, which do not normally express major histocompatibility complex (MHC) class II molecules, do so in Graves' thyroiditis [35], and having noted the role class II molecule-expressing antigen-presenting cells play in the activation of helper T lymphocytes, Bottazzo and coworkers [36] suggested the general theory that cells which have been aberrantly induced to express class II molecules initiate autoimmune responses by presenting their own surface constituents to reactive T lymphocytes. There have subsequently been numerous observations that the targets of autoimmune and inflammatory responses express class II molecules [37]. These examples include several ophthalmic conditions, such as corneal transplant rejection [38], uveitis [39], experimental autoimmune uveoretinitis [40], retinitis pigmentosa [41], and proliferative vitreoretinopathy [42]. That class II molecule expression may play an important role in the initiation of such phenomena is suggested by the ability of antibodies to class II molecules to protect against experimental autoimmune uveitis [43]. Of particular relevance in attempts to understand the events leading to lymphocytic proliferation in the lacrimal (and salivary) glands is the fact that class II molecule expression is uniformly observed on salivary epithelial cells of Sjögren's syndrome patients [44, 45]. Lacrimal epithelial cells can be induced to express class II molecules and, in a survey of cadaver donor lacrimal glands, the numbers of epithelial cells expressing class II molecules generally increased with the number of lymphocytes infiltrating the gland [46]. It may be noted that class II molecule expression has not been uniformly detected in Sjögren's lacrimal glands [10].

A number of autoimmune diseases map to the HLA-DR region of chromosome 6, and particular class II MHC haplotypes are frequently observed in certain autoimmune diseases [47, 48]. HLA-DR2 and -DR3 are very strongly correlated with the production of antibodies to Ro(SS-A) and La(SS-B) in Sjögren's syndrome [49, 50]. Recent work focuses particular attention on the specific extended haplotype DR3, DR52a, DQA4, and DQB2 [51, 52]. One likely explanation is that the haplotypes which confer high risks are those which have affinities for the immunogenic peptides generated in potential target cells.

Macrophages and the other specialized antigen-presenting cells typically use class II molecules to present antigens to helper (CD4$^+$) T lymphocytes. However, there is also a significant precedent for the use of class II molecules in the activation of cytotoxic-suppressor (CD8$^+$) T lymphocytes [53], so that aberrant expression of class II molecules could, conceivably, contribute to the vigorous CD8$^+$ lymphocytic infiltration of AIDS adenopathy as well as to the more benign lymphocytic proliferation observed in the aging lacrimal and salivary glands.

Studies with lymphoblastoid cells have provided considerable evidence to support the proposition that class II molecules can mediate the presentation of endogenous as well as exogenous antigens [54–56]. There is also a growing number of examples of nonlymphoblastoid cells that have been demonstrated to present antigens and activate T lymphocytes effectively after they have been induced to express class II molecules. These include thyroid follicular cells from Graves' thyroiditis patients, which activate co-cultured autologous thyroid lymphocytes in a class II molecule–restricted fashion [57]. Rat lymph nodes contain lymphocytes that can be activated in MHC class II–restricted fashion by a continuous line of rat thyroid follicular cells, which are immature cells of the helper subset that, presumably, have not undergone deletion in the thymus [58]. Cultured rat retinal pigment epithelial cells that have been induced to express class II molecules by stimulation with interferon gamma are able to induce T-cell proliferation in vitro by processing and presenting S antigen [59].

It should be noted that there are also instances in which inappropriate class II molecule expression has failed to induce the lymphocytic proliferation and tissue destruction reminiscent of autoimmunity. Transgenic mice constructed to express class II molecules on pancreatic islet cells may [60] or may not [61] develop islet cell atrophy and insulin-dependent diabetes, but they generally fail to exhibit lymphocytic proliferation characteristic of insulin-dependent diabetes mellitus. In other instances, class II molecule–expressing nonlymphoid cells appear to suppress rather than induce T-lymphocyte activation [62].

■ Importance of Accessory Signals for T-Cell Activation

It is now apparent that T-cell activation depends on the conjunction of two signals, a signal mediated through the T-cell receptor and triggered by class II molecule–mediated antigen presentation, and an accessory (or second) signal carried by soluble mediators, such as interleukin 2 (IL2) [63]. Fibroblasts that have been induced to express class II molecules can activate T lymphocytes only if IL2 or other factors are continuously present, either added exogenously or released by cocultured class II molecule–negative endothelial cells [64]. IL2 usually is included in lymphocyte–epithelial cell coculture systems to induce epithelial cell class II molecule expression, and it now appears likely that this cytokine plays a second role as the accessory signal for in vitro T-cell activation. A failure to satisfy the requirement for appropriate accessory signals may account for the failures of class II molecule transgenic animals to develop overt autoimmune disease.

■ Antigen Processing and Intracellular Traffic of Class II Molecules

The theory that aberrantly expressed class II molecules mediate the presentation of autoantigens was proposed at a time when the phenomena of antigen processing and presentation in the specialized antigen-presenting cells were incompletely understood. The current picture of antigen processing and presentation can be summarized as follows [65, 66]: Foreign proteins are internalized, by fluid-phase endocytosis or by receptor-mediated endocytosis [67], to a compartment that contains proteolytic enzymes, most notably the aspartyl protease, cathepsin D, and the thiol protease, cathepsin B [68, 69]. This endosome provides a milieu that is sufficiently acidic to permit the cathepsins to be catalytically active, so that proteins entering it are converted to peptide fragments and free amino acids. Class II molecules also enter the protease-containing endocytic compartment [70, 71], at least during their first pass through the membrane assembly pathway [72] and, in some cell types, during their subsequent recycling to and from the surface membrane [73, 74]. The newly synthesized class II molecules emerge from the endoplasmic reticulum associated with invariant chain, which association probably remains intact until the complex reaches the endosomes [75]. Invariant chain is not tightly bound to the class II molecule, and its replacement by peptide fragments appears to increase the stability of the heterodimeric class II molecule and to accelerate its translocation to the cell surface membrane. It appears that "empty" class II molecules may also reach the cell surface [76, 77]. Alternatively, the nature of the peptides bound to class II molecules may be determined by mass action [78].

How Lacrimal Acinar Cells May Mimic Specialized Antigen-Presenting Cells

Werdelin [79] has suggested that cellular proteins may be processed and presented as autoantigens if they enter the normal pathway for protein degradation in a cell that expresses class II molecules. It now is possible to suggest a specific hypothesis for how closely epithelial cells may mimic the specialized antigen-presenting cells when they begin to express class II molecules.

Intracellular Pools of Plasma Membrane Constituents

It has been known since the work of Herzog and Farquhar [80] that after secretory vesicles fuse with the apical plasma membrane to release their contents in stimulated exocytosis, the vesicle membrane constituents are endocytically retrieved and recycled. There is also considerable evidence for extensive recycling traffic between endosomal compartments and the basal-lateral plasma membranes of lacrimal acinar cells. Fluid-phase markers, such as horseradish peroxidase, when injected into the circulation, appear in endosomal structures in rat and guinea pig lacrimal acinar cells, and this endocytic process is accelerated by secretagogues [81]. Lacrimal acinar cells contain large intracellular pools of all plasma membrane constituents that have been examined to date [82–84], including muscarinic cholinergic receptors and beta-adrenergic receptors [85], which mediate the acinar cell's response to autonomic secretomotor stimulation and Na,K-ATPase pump units, Na/H antiporters, and Cl/HCO_3 antiporters, which are key components of the cell's mechanism of acinar fluid secretion [86]. When lacrimal gland acinar cells are stimulated with the cholinergic agonist carbachol, Na,K-ATPase pump units are mobilized from the intracellular pool and translocated to the basal-lateral plasma membranes [87–89]. The cellular rationale for this redistribution is that additional pumps are needed to drive an increased rate of transepithelial salt secretion. Muscarinic cholinergic receptors also appear to participate to some extent in the membrane traffic, as the intracellular pool of receptors becomes significantly depleted, while the plasma membrane–expressed pool appears to increase slightly [90]. The rationale for this phenomenon may be to allow the cell to secrete fluid at a sustained rate in response to persistent secretomotor stimulation.

The organization of the intracellular pools of plasma membrane constituents, and of the traffic between them, is beginning to emerge. Distinct early endosomes appear to mediate retrieval of secretory vesicle membrane constituents from the apical plasma membranes and to mediate fluid-phase endocytosis from the basal-lateral membranes [91]. An analogy to other types of epithelial cells suggests that the lacrimal acinar cell may also contain a late endosomal compartment that is in fluid-phase communication with both the apical and basal-lateral early endosomes [92]. Communication between the apically and basal-laterally oriented recycling pathways should be a critical feature of the transcytotic secretion of dimeric IgA [93]. Such communication probably also allows the acinar cells to internalize prolactin from the interstitium and package it into secretory vesicles for regulated secretion [2].

Recent experiments with isolated rabbit lacrimal gland acinar cells substantiate the existence of distinct early and late endosomal compartments. Carbachol accelerates endocytic uptake of the fluid-phase marker Lucifer yellow. Carbachol also increases the cell's steady-state content of the fluid-phase marker, suggesting that, in addition to accelerating traffic between the plasma membrane and an early endosome, it also activates traffic between the early endosome and a late endosome. That the bulk of the endocytic traffic proceeds mainly via the early basal-lateral endosome rather than the early apical endosome is indicated by the results of surface labeling experiments (discussed later) and by the observation that fluid-phase endocytosis is more sensitive to carbachol than is secretory protein release. Carbachol-dependent traffic to the late endosome stops when the incubation temperature is reduced from 37° to 18°C. By exploiting this temperature block, it is possible to label selectively the early basal-lateral endosome or to label both the early and late endosomes with fluid-phase markers, so that their membranes can be identified in subcellular fractionation analyses. Such analyses indicate that the recruitable reserve of Na,K-ATPase pump units is localized in the late endosome (JP Gierow and AK Mircheff, unpublished observations). Thus, activation of traffic between the late and early basal-lateral endosome is accompanied by translocation of a population of Na,K-ATPase pump units from the late endosome to the basal-lateral membrane recycling traffic.

Traffic between the basal-lateral plasma membrane and the early basal-lateral endosome is remarkably rapid [94]. If a suspension of acinar cells is chilled to 4°C to stop membrane traffic, then labeled by sequential incubations with sulfo-N-hydroxysuccinimidyl-biotin (sulfo-N-HS-biotin) and either avidin–Lucifer yellow or avidin-ferritin conjugate, the label can be detected at the plasma membranes as long as the cells are maintained at

4°C. Most of the label is internalized when the cells are warmed to 37°C. When cells are allowed to internalize surface biotinyl groups, then exposed to avidin–Lucifer yellow conjugate at 37°C, they take up avidin–Lucifer yellow in a saturable, time-dependent fashion, indicating that the internalized plasma membrane recycles back to the cell surface. Moreover, this recycling traffic is accelerated severalfold by stimulation with carbachol.

The recycling traffic of typical basal-lateral membrane constituents appears to carry along with it a turnover flux of class II molecules [95]. Surface-expressed class II molecules can be labeled by sequential incubations at 4°C with the monoclonal antibody 2C4, biotinylated goat antimouse IgG, and avidin-ferritin conjugate. The ferritin label is rapidly internalized on warming to 37°C. However, the cells fail to accumulate large amounts of monoclonal antibody 2C4 during prolonged incubations at 37°C, suggesting that class II molecules are degraded after they have been internalized from the cell surface. The steady-state intracellular pool of class II molecules—detected by postembedding labeling with monoclonal antibody 2C4, biotinylated goat antimouse IgG, and avidin-gold conjugate—remains large, and the cells continue to internalize class II molecules from their surface membranes.

Our working hypothesis for the intracellular traffic of class II molecules can be summarized as follows: Newly synthesized class II molecules move sequentially from the Golgi complex to the transreticular Golgi network, the late endosome, and the early basal-lateral endosome. After being internalized from the plasma membrane and returned to the early basal-lateral endosome, class II molecules are directed to lysosomes to be degraded.

Cathepsin D and Cathepsin B

Additional experiments indicate that lacrimal gland acinar cells contain cathepsin D and cathepsin B catalytic activities. The subcellular localization of cathepsin B has been surveyed. Immunogold cytochemical studies using a sheep antibody to human cathepsin B suggest that this proteolytic enzyme is present in lysosomes and also, in even larger amounts, in secretory vesicles (K-H Park and RL Wood, unpublished data). Subcellular fractionation analyses indicate that smaller, but still measurable, amounts of cathepsin B are present in the endosomal membranes (JP Gierow, S Rafisolyman, and AK Mircheff, unpublished data). This distribution pattern is similar to those exhibited by other lysosomal enzymes, which may enter the endosomes before they are recaptured and packaged for delivery to the lysosomes [96].

The flux of class II molecules through endosomes that contain cathepsins would seem to set the stage for the lacrimal acinar cell to function as an antigen-presenting cell. It is probable that virtually any protein the cell synthesizes may enter the endosomes and become subject to catheptic processing, because the process of autophagy in exocrine acinar cells delivers samples of the cytoplasm to the endomembrane system at a point that appears to correspond to the late endosome [97]. For cytoplasmic proteins to be hydrolyzed by endosomal cathepsins, the autophagic vesicles in which they are contained would have to be lysed. In this context it is noteworthy that, like other secretory cells, lacrimal acinar cells contain membrane-associated phospholipases that are activated by secretomotor stimulation. If these phospholipases are associated with endosomal membranes as well as the basal-lateral plasma membranes—a likely proposition, as all the plasma membrane constituents that have been studied so far have such complex subcellular distributions—then they would be situated where they could disrupt autophagocytic vesicles within the endosomes. That traffic through the endomembrane system underlies the generation and presentation of autoantigens is suggested by the report that sera from Sjögren's syndrome patients contain anti–Golgi complex IgG [98]. It has also been reported that infection of cultured human kidney cells with adenovirus, CMV, and EBV causes the La(SS-B) antigen to be expressed at higher-than-normal levels and to redistribute from the nucleus to the cytoplasm and, in some cases, the plasma membrane [99]; such changes may augment the flux of La(SS-B) into the endomembrane system, increasing the likelihood that it will be subjected to catheptic processing and class II molecule–mediated presentation.

Effects of Interferon Gamma and Other Factors

The lacrimal acinar cell would not normally function as an autoantigen-presenting cell because it does not normally express class II molecules. The most prominent candidate among the factors that may induce class II molecule expression is interferon gamma released during local inflammatory responses [36]. Infection by EBV or other viruses may also promote class II molecule expression independently of the presence or absence of interferon gamma [100]. In addition, it seems plausible that interferon gamma and other cytokines that enter the circulation during infections and autoimmune processes in other organs may reach the lacrimal glands in levels high enough to promote class II molecule expression. The observation that thyroid-stimulating hormone (TSH) is a potent inducer of class II molecule expression by thyroid follicular cells [101] raises the additional possibility that the hormones and neurotransmitters which acutely regulate lacrimal secretion may, if present at elevated levels or for sustained times, also influence acinar cell class II molecule expression. There is already some indication that carbachol enhances class II molecule expression by lacrimal acinar cells ([46]; also RL Wood, JP Gierow, and AK Mircheff, unpublished data).

Segregation Mechanisms

Physiological circumstances may influence the spectrum of peptide fragments generated within the endomembrane system and, therefore, the peptides that may be presented to potentially autoreactive T lymphocytes. The fact that the normal response to cholinergic stimulation triggers the selective release of reserve Na,K-ATPase pump units from the late endosome implies the operation of a segregation mechanism that retains other membrane constituents within the late endosome. A breakdown of this segregation may release new constituents into the membrane recycling system. In in vitro studies of fluid-phase endocytosis, increasing the concentration of carbachol from its optimum of 10 μmolar to the supramaximal value of 1 mmolar appears to perturb traffic between the early and late endosomes [102], suggesting that during sustained excessive stimulation, unusually large amounts of newly synthesized proteins may accumulate in the late endosomes. Removal of the stimulus might then release a flood of membrane constituents and intracisternal products, which overwhelm the segregation mechanisms. As in other types of epithelial cells [103, 104], excessive stimulation also induces the formation of aqueous vacuoles in the apical cytoplasm (RL Wood, JP Gierow, and AK Mircheff, unpublished observations). These vacuoles appear to result from fusion of secretory vesicles with one another and with other structures of the endomembrane system.

Outcome of Class II Molecule Induction

The outcome of class II molecule–mediated autoantigen presentation depends on several factors, including the presence of reactive helper T lymphocytes and the availability of accessory signals that will determine whether engagement of the T-cell receptor leads to activation or anergy. Several accessory signal molecules may be present in the lacrimal interstitium. Stepkowski and coworkers [105] have reported that lacrimal acinar cells in primary culture produce an IL2-like molecule, and Liu and colleagues [106] have found that lacrimal glands contain a factor that potentiates the proliferation of activated lymphocytes. It is also noteworthy that prolactin, which accumulates within lacrimal acinar cells, has been implicated in both normal immune and autoimmune responses [107]. As noted previously, the lacrimal duct epithelium produces EGF, and production of fibroblast growth factor has been reported as well [108]. Additionally, autonomic and sensory nerve fibers terminating in the lacrimal glands release a rich variety of neurotransmitters and neuropeptides, including several (such as substance P, calcitonin gene-related peptide, vasoactive intestinal peptide [109, 110], and enkephalins [111]) that are believed to modulate lymphocytic activity.

Over time, a number of events occur that may lead lacrimal acinar cells to begin expressing class II molecules, and so it is not uncommon to observe class II molecule expression on epithelial cells in the lacrimal glands of aged individuals [46]. There is ample reason to suspect that the induction of class II molecule expression and lapses of normal endomembrane segregation mechanisms may occur more frequently in women than in men. The lacrimal glands are part of a servomechanism designed to keep the ocular surface adequately lubricated. The decline in secretory capacity that occurs with loss of hormonal support would, therefore, be predicted to cause an increase in the intensity and duration of autonomic secretomotor stimulation to the gland. Such increased stimulation may enhance class II molecule expression, accelerate autophagy [112], and increase the likelihood of events that override normal endomembrane segregation mechanisms [102]. We contend that in most individuals, class II molecule–mediated autoantigen presentation leads to helper T-lymphocyte responses that are counterbalanced by suppressor responses. The gradually progressive accumulation of lymphocytes through such interactions may account for the normal pattern of lymphocytic infiltration of the lacrimal glands. In other circumstances—perhaps determined by excessive pressure of autoantigen presentation by especially effective class II molecules, a particularly conducive milieu of accessory signals, production of growth-stimulating autocrine factors and inadequate suppressor mechanisms—proliferation of helper T lymphocytes and B cells may proceed without effective restraint, crossing the threshold between normal autoimmunity and autoimmune disease.

Work in the authors' laboratories has been supported by National Institutes of Health grants EY05801 and EY09405; grants from the Wright Foundation (Los Angeles, CA), the Doheny Eye Institute (Los Angeles, CA), and University of Southern California School of Medicine Biomedical Research Support Grants; a postdoctoral fellowship award from Fight for Sight—Prevent Blindness, Inc. (Schaumberg, IL); a research fellowship award from the Sjögren's Syndrome Foundation, Inc. (Port Washington, NY); and a gift from Dr. Ronald H. Akashi (Monterey Park, CA).

■ References

1. Frey WH, Nelson JD, Frisk ML, Elde RP. Prolactin immunoreactivity in human tears and lacrimal gland: possible implications for tear production. In: Holly FJ, ed. The preocular tear film in health, disease, and contact lens wear. Lubbock: Dry Eye Institute, 1986:798–807
2. Wood RL, Park K-H, Gierow JP, Mircheff AK. Immunogold localization of prolactin in acinar cells of lacrimal gland. In: Sullivan DA, ed. The lacrimal gland, tear film, and dry eye syndromes. New York: Plenum, 1994:in press

3. van Setten GB, Tervo K, Virtanen I, et al. Immunohistochemical demonstration of epidermal growth factor in the lacrimal and submandibular glands of rats. Acta Ophthalmol (Copenh) 1990;68:477–480
4. Franklin RM, Kenyon KR, Tomasi TB. Immunohistologic studies of human lacrimal gland: localization of immunoglobulins, secretory component, and lactoferrin. J Immunol 1973;110:984–992
5. Wieczorek R, Jakobiec FA, Sacks EH, Knowles M. The immunoarchitecture of the normal human lacrimal gland. Ophthalmology 1988;95:100–109
6. Gudmundsson OG, Benediktsson H, Olafdottir K. T-lymphocyte subsets in the human lacrimal gland. Acta Ophthalmol (Copenh) 1988;66:19–23
7. Sjögren H, Bloch KJ. Keratoconjunctivitis sicca and the Sjögren syndrome. Surv Ophthalmol 1971;16:145–159
8. Williamson J, Gibson AAM, Wilson T, et al. Histology of the lacrimal gland in keratoconjunctivitis sicca. Br J Ophthalmol 1973;57:852
9. Pflugfelder SC, Wilhelmus KR, Osato MS, et al. The autoimmune nature of aqueous tear deficiency. Ophthalmology 1986;93:1513–1517
10. Pepose JS, Akata RF, Pflugfelder SC, Voigt W. Mononuclear cell phenotypes and immunoglobulin gene rearrangements in lacrimal gland biopsies from patients with Sjögren's syndrome. Ophthalmology 1990;97:1599–1605
11. Gumpel JM, Hobbs JR. Serum immune globulins in Sjögren's syndrome. Ann Rheum Dis 1970;29:681–683
12. Fox RI, Robinson C, Curd J, et al. First international symposium on Sjögren's syndrome: suggested criteria for classification. Scand J Rheumatol 1986;suppl 61:28–30
13. Forstot JZ, Forstot SL, Greer RO, Tan EM. The incidence of Sjögren's sicca complex in a population of patients with keratoconjunctivitis sicca. Arthritis Rheum 1982;25:156–160
14. Strickland RW, Tesar JT, Berne BH, et al. The frequency of sicca syndrome in an elderly female population. J Rheumatol 1987;14:766–771
15. Markusse HM, Hogeweg M, Swaak AJG, et al. Ophthalmological examinations of patients with primary Sjögren's syndrome selected from a rheumatology practice. Br J Rheumatol 1992;31:473–476
16. Segerberg-Konttinen M. Focal adenitis in lacrimal and salivary glands. Scand J Rheumatol 1988;17:379–385
17. Damato BE, Allan D, Murray SB, Lee WR. Senile atrophy of the human lacrimal gland: the contribution of chronic inflammatory disease. Br J Ophthalmol 1984;68:674–680
18. Rose NE, Griffin DE. Virus-induced autoimmunity. In: Talal N, ed. Molecular autoimmunity. San Diego: Academic, 1991:247–272
19. Burns JC. Persistent cytomegalovirus infection—the etiology of Sjögren's syndrome. Med Hypotheses 1983;10:451–460
20. Whittingham S, McNeilage J, MacKay IR. Primary Sjögren's syndrome after infectious mononucleosis. Ann Intern Med 1985;102:490–493
21. Pflugfelder SC, Roussel TJ, Culbertson WW. Primary Sjögren's syndrome after infectious mononucleosis. JAMA 1987;257:1049–1050
22. Fox RI, Pearson G, Vaughn JH. Detection of Epstein-Barr virus–associated antigens and DNA in salivary gland biopsies from patients with Sjögren's syndrome. J Immunol 1986;137:3162–3168
23. Mariette X, Gozlan J, Clerc D, et al. Detection of Epstein-Barr virus DNA by *in situ* hybridization and polymerase chain reaction in salivary gland biopsy specimens from patients with Sjögren's syndrome. Am J Med 1991;90:286–294
24. Pflugfelder SC, Crouse C, Pereira I, Atherton S. Amplification of Epstein-Barr virus genomic sequences in blood cells, lacrimal glands, and tears from primary Sjögren's syndrome patients. Ophthalmology 1990;97:976–984

25. Pflugfelder SC, Tseng SCG, Pepose JS, et al. Epstein-Barr virus infection and immunologic dysfunction in patients with aqueous tear deficiency. Ophthalmology 1990;97:313–323
26. Crouse CA, Pflugfelder SC, Cleary T, et al. Detection of Epstein-Barr genomes in normal human lacrimal glands. J Clin Microbiol 1990;28:1026–1032
27. Deacon LM, Shattles WG, Mathews JB, et al. Frequency of EBV DNA detection in Sjögren's syndrome. Am J Med 1992;92:453–454
28. Fox RI, Kang H-I. Pathogenesis of Sjögren's syndrome. Rheum Dis Clin North Am 1992;18:517–538
29. Garry RF, Fermin CD, Hart D, et al. Detection of a human intracisternal A-type retroviral particle antigenically related to HIV. Science 1990;250:1127–1129
30. Lucca JA, Farris RL, Bielory L, Caputo AR. Keratoconjunctivitis sicca in male patients infected with immunodeficiency virus type 1. Ophthalmology 1990;97:1008–1010
31. Itescu S, Brancato LJ, Buxbaum J, et al. A diffuse infiltrative CD8 lymphocytosis syndrome in human immunodeficiency virus (HIV) infection: a host immune response associated with HLA-DR5. Ann Intern Med 1990;122:3–10
32. Talal N, Flescher E, Dang H. Are endogenous retroviruses involved in human autoimmune disease? J Autoimmun 1992;5(suppl A):61–66
33. Miyasaka N, Yamaoka K, Sato K, et al. An analysis of polyclonal B cell activation in Sjögren's syndrome. Characterization of B cell lines spontaneously established from the peripheral blood. Scand J Rheumatol 1986;61:123–126
34. Takei M, Dang H, Dauphinee MJ, Talal N. Autostimulatory growth factors produced by Sjögren's syndrome B cell lines. Clin Immunol Immunopathol 1989;53:123–135
35. Hanafusa T, Pujol-Borrell R, Choviato L, et al. Aberrant expression of HLA-DR antigen on thyrocytes in Graves' disease. Relevance for autoimmunity. Lancet 1983;2:1112–1115
36. Bottazzo GF, Pujol-Borrell R, Hanafusa T. Role of aberrant HLA-DR expression and antigen presentation in induction of endocrine autoimmunity. Lancet 1983;2:1115–1118
37. Bottazzo GF, Todd I, Mirakian R, et al. Organ-specific autoimmunity: a 1986 update. Immunol Rev 1986;94:137–169
38. Pepose JS, Gerdner KM, Nestor MS, et al. Detection of HLA Class I and Class II antigens in rejected human corneal allografts. Ophthalmology 1985;92:1480–1484
39. Chan C-C, Detrick B, Nussenblatt RB, et al. HLA-DR antigens on retinal pigment epithelial cells from patients with uveitis. Arch Ophthalmol 1986;104:725–729
40. Chan C-C, Caspi RR, Roberge FG, Nussenblatt RB. Dynamics of experimental autoimmune uveoretinitis induced by adoptive transfers of S-antigen-specific T cell line. Invest Ophthalmol Vis Sci 1988;29:411–418
41. Detrick B, Rodrigues M, Chan C-C, et al. Expression of HLA-DR antigen on retinal pigment epithelial cells in retinitis pigmentosa. Am J Ophthalmol 1986;101:584–590
42. Baudouin C, Brignole F, Bayle J, et al. Class II histocompatibility antigen expression by cellular components of vitreous and subretinal fluid in proliferative vitreoretinopathy. Invest Ophthalmol Vis Sci 1991;32:2065–2072
43. Rao NA, Atalla L, Linker-Israeli M, et al. Suppression of experimental uveitis in rats by anti-I-A antibodies. Invest Ophthalmol Vis Sci 1989;30:2348–2355
44. Fox RI, Bumol T, Fantozzi R, et al. Expression of histocompatibility antigen HLA-DR by salivary gland epithelial cells in Sjögren's syndrome. Arthritis Rheum 1986;29:1105–1111
45. Franco A, Valesini G, Barnaba V, et al. Class II MHC antigen expression on

epithelial cells of salivary glands from patients with Sjögren's syndrome. Clin Exp Rheumatol 1987;5:199–203
46. Mircheff AK, Gierow JP, Lambert RW, et al. Class II antigen expression by lacrimal epithelial cells. An updated working hypothesis for antigen presentation by epithelial cells. Invest Ophthalmol Vis Sci 1991;32:3202–3310
47. Scholz SG, Albert ED. HLA and autoimmune diseases. In: Bigazzi PE, Wick G, Wicher K, eds. Organ-specific autoimmunity. New York: Marcel Dekker, 1990: 11–23
48. Todd JA, Acha-Orbea H, Bell JI, et al. A molecular basis for MHC Class II–associated autoimmunity. Science 1988;240:1003–2009
49. Wilson WW, Provost TT, Bias WB, et al. Sjögren's syndrome. Influence of multiple HLA-D region alloantigens on clinical and serologic expression. Arthritis Rheum 1984;27:1245–1253
50. Foster H, Walker D, Charles P, et al. Association of DR3 with susceptibility to and severity of primary Sjögren's syndrome in a family study. Br J Rheumatol 1992;31:309–314
51. Harley JB, Reichlin M, Arnett FC, et al. Gene interaction at HLA-DQ enhances autoantibody production in primary Sjögren's syndrome. Science 1986;232: 1145–1147
52. Fei HM, Kang H, Scharf S, et al. Specific HLA-DQA and HLA-DRB1 alleles confer susceptibility to Sjögren's syndrome and autoantibody production. J Clin Lab Anal 1991;5:382–391
53. Muller D, Koller BH, Whitton JL, et al. LCMV-specific, class II restricted cytotoxic T cells in β_2-microglobulin-deficient mice. Science 1992;255:1576–1578
54. Jaraquemada D, Marti M, Long EO. An endogenous processing pathway in vaccinia virus–infected cells for presentation of cytoplasmic antigens to Class II–restricted T cells. J Exp Med 1990;172:947–954
55. Nuchtern JG, Biddison WE, Klausner RD. Class II MHC molecules can use the endogenous pathway of antigen presentation. Nature 1990;343:74–76
56. Martin A, Magnusson RP, Kendler DL, et al. Endogenous antigen presentation by autoantigen-transfected Epstein-Barr virus–lymphoblastoid cells. J Clin Invest 1993;91:1567–1574
57. Grubeck-Loebenstein B, Londei M, Greenall C, et al. Pathogenic relevance of HLA Class II expressing thyroid follicular cells in nontoxic goiter and in Graves' disease. J Clin Invest 1988;81:1608–1614
58. Kimura H, Davies T. Thyroid specific T cell lines in the normal Wistar rat. Clin Immunol Immunopathol 1991;58:195–206
59. Percopo CM, Hooks JJ, Shinohara T, et al. Cytokine-mediated activation of a neuronal retinal resident cell provokes antigen presentation. J Immunol 1990;145: 4101–4107
60. Sarvetnick N, Liggitt D, Pitts S, et al. Insulin-dependent diabetes mellitus induced in transgenic mice by ectopic expression of Class II MHC and interferon-gamma. Cell 1988;52:773–782
61. Böhme J, Haslins K, Stecha P, et al. Transgenic mice with I-A on islet cells are normoglycemic but immunologically intolerant. Science 1989;244:1179–1183
62. Caspi RR, Roberge FG, Nussenblatt RB. Organ-resident, nonlymphoid cells suppress proliferation of autoimmune T-helper lymphocytes. Science 1987;237: 1029–1032
63. Mueller DL, Jenkins MK, Schwartz RH. Clonal expansion versus functional clonal inactivation: a costimulatory signalling pathway determines the outcome of T cell antigen receptor occupancy. Ann Rev Immunol 1989;7:445–480
64. Geppert TD, Lipsky PE. Dissection of defective antigen presentation by interferon-γ-treated fibroblasts. J Immunol 1987;138:385–392

65. Unanue ER, Cerottini J-C. Antigen presentation. FASEB J 1989;3:2496–2502
66. Brodsky FM, Guagliardi LE. The cell biology of antigen processing and presentation. Ann Rev Immunol 1991;9:707–744
67. Lanzavecchia A. Receptor-mediated antigen uptake and its effect on antigen presentation to Class II–restricted T lymphocytes. Ann Rev Immunol 1990;8:773–793
68. Diment S. Different roles for thiol and aspartyl proteases in antigen presentation of ovalbumin. J Immunol 1990;145:417–422
69. van der Drift ACM, van Noort JM, Krüse J. Catheptic processing of protein antigens: enzymatic and molecular aspects. Semin Immunol 1990;2:255–271
70. Guagliardi LE, Koppelman B, Blum JS, et al. Co-localization of molecules involved in antigen processing and presentation in an early endocytic compartment. Nature 1990;343:133–139
71. Harding CV, Geuze HJ. Class II molecules are present in macrophage lysosomes and phagolysosomes that function in the phagocytic processing of *Listeria monocytogenes* for presentation to T cells. J Cell Biol 1992;1190:531–542
72. Neffjes JJ, Stollorz V, Peters PJ, et al. The biosynthetic pathway of MHC Class II but not Class I molecules intersects the endocytic route. Cell 1990;61:171–183
73. Aragnol D, Malissen B, Schiff C, et al. Endocytosis of MHC molecules by B cell–B lymphoma and B cell–T lymphoma hybrids. J Immunol 1986;137:3347–3353
74. Reid PA, Watts C. Cycling of cell-surface MHC glycoproteins through primaquine-sensitive intracellular compartments. Nature 1990;346:655–657
75. Pieters J, Horstmann H, Bakke O, et al. Intracellular transport and localization of major histocompatibility complex Class II molecules and invariant chain. J Cell Biol 1991;115:1213–1223
76. Germain RN, Hendrix LR. MHC Class II structure, occupancy and surface expression determined by post-endoplasmic reticulum antigen binding. Nature 1991;353:134–139
77. Sette S, Ceman S, Kubo T, et al. Invariant chain peptides in most HLA-DR molecules of an antigen processing mutant. Science 1992;258:1801–1804
78. Gautam AM, Glynn P. Competition between foreign and self proteins in antigen presentation. J Immunol 1990;144:1177–1180
79. Werdelin O. Autoantigen processing and the mechanisms of tolerance to self. In: Bigassi PE, Wick G, Wicher K, eds. Organ specific autoimmunity. New York: Marcel Dekker, 1990:1–9
80. Herzog V, Farquhar MG. Luminal membrane retrieved after exocytosis reaches most Golgi cisternae in secretory cells. Proc Natl Acad Sci USA 1977;74:5073–5077
81. Oliver C. Endocytic pathways at the lateral and basal surfaces of exocrine acinar cells. J Cell Biol 1982;95:154–161
82. Mircheff AK, Lu CC. A map of membrane populations isolated from rat exorbital gland. Am J Physiol 1984;247:G651–G661
83. Yiu SC, Wood RL, Mircheff AK. Analytic fractionation of acini from rat lacrimal gland. Invest Ophthalmol Vis Sci 1990;31:2437–2447
84. Bradley ME, Azuma K, McDonough AA, et al. Surface and intracellular pools of Na,K-ATPase catalytic- and immuno-activities in rat exorbital lacrimal gland. Exp Eye Res 1993;57:403–413
85. Bradley ME, Lambert RW, Lambert RW, et al. Isolation and subcellular fractionation analysis of acini from rabbit lacrimal glands. Invest Ophthalmol Vis Sci 1992;33:2951–2965
86. Lambert RW, Bradley ME, Mircheff AK. pH-sensitive anion exchanger in rat lacrimal acinar cells. Am J Physiol 1991;260:G517–G523
87. Yiu SC, Lambert RW, Bradley ME, et al. Stimulation-associated redistribution of Na,K-ATPase in rat lacrimal gland. J Membr Biol 1988;102:185–194

88. Yiu SC, Lambert RW, Tortoriello PJ, Mircheff AK. Secretagogue-induced redistributions of Na,K-ATPase in rat lacrimal acini. Invest Ophthalmol Vis Sci 1991;32: 2976–2984
89. Lambert RW, Maves CA, Mircheff AK. Carbachol-induced increase of Na$^+$/H$^+$ antiport and recruitment of Na$^+$,K$^+$-ATPase in rabbit lacrimal acini. Curr Eye Res 1993;12:539–551
90. Bradley ME, Peters CL, Lambert RW, et al. Subcellular distribution of muscarinic acetylcholine receptors in rat exorbital lacrimal gland. Invest Ophthalmol Vis Sci 1990;31:977–986
91. Oliver C, Hand AR. Membrane retrieval in exocrine acinar cells. Methods Cell Biol 1982;23:429–444
92. Parton RG, Prydz K, Bomsel M, et al. Meeting of the apical and basolateral endocytic pathways of the Madin-Darby canine kidney cell in late endosomes. J Cell Biol 1989;109:3259–3272
93. Schaerer E, Neutra MR, Kraehenbuhl J-P. Molecular and cellular mechanisms involved in transepithelial transport. J Membr Biol 1991;123:93–103
94. Lambert RW, Maves CA, Gierow JP, et al. Plasma membrane internalization and recycling in rabbit lacrimal acinar cells. Invest Ophthalmol Vis Sci 1993;34: 305–316
95. Mircheff AK, Gierow JP, Wood RL. Traffic of Class II MHC molecules in rabbit lacrimal gland acinar cells. Invest Ophthalmol Vis Sci 1993;34s:821
96. Ludwig T, Griffiths G, Hoflack B. Distribution of newly synthesized lysosomal enzymes in the endocytic pathway of normal rat kidney cells. J Cell Biol 1991;115: 1561–1572
97. Tooze J, Hollinshead M, Ludwig T, et al. In exocrine pancreas, the basolateral endocytic pathway converges with the autophagic pathway immediately after the early endosome. J Cell Biol 1990;111:329–345
98. Blaschek MA, Pennec YL, Simitzis AM, et al. Anti-Golgi complex autoantibodies in patients with primary Sjögren's syndrome. Scand J Rheumatol 1988;17:291–296
99. Baboonian C, Venables PJW, Booth J, et al. Virus infection induces redistribution and membrane localization of the nuclear antigen La (SS-B): a possible mechanism for autoimmunity. Clin Exp Immunol 1989;78:454–459
100. Issekutz T, Cho E, Geha RS. Antigen presentation by human B cells: T cell proliferation induced by Epstein Barr virus B lymphoblastoid cells. J Immunol 1982; 129:1446–1450
101. Todd J, Pujol-Borrell R, Hammond LJ, et al. Enhancement of HLA Class II expression by thyroid stimulating hormone. Clin Exp Immunol 1987;69:524–531
102. Gierow JP, Wood RL, Mircheff AK. Endocytosis and exocytosis in rabbit lacrimal gland acinar cells. In: Sullivan DA, ed. The lacrimal gland, tear film, and dry eye syndromes. New York: Plenum, 1994:in press
103. Mills JW, Quinton PM. Formation of stimulus-induced vacuoles in serous cells of tracheal submucosal glands. Am J Physiol 1981;241:C18–C24
104. Watanabe O, Baccino FM, Steer ML, Meldolesi J. Supramaximal caerulein stimulation and ultrastructure of rat pancreatic acinar cells: early morphological changes during development of experimental pancreatitis. Am J Physiol 1984;246: G457–G467
105. Stepkowski SM, Li T, Franklin R. Interleukin-2 like molecule produced by acinar cells in lacrimal gland regulates local immune response. Invest Ophthalmol Vis Sci 1993;34S:1486
106. Liu SH, Zhou D-Z, Franklin RM. Lacrimal gland-derived lymphocyte proliferation potentiating factor. Invest Ophthalmol Vis Sci 1993;34:650–657
107. Buskila D, Sukenik S, Shoenfeld Y. The possible role of prolactin in autoimmunity. Am J Reprod Immunol 1991;26:118–123
108. Wilson SE, Lloyd SA, Kennedy RH. Basic fibroblast growth factor (FGFb) and

epidermal growth factor (EGF) receptor messenger RNA production in human lacrimal gland. Invest Ophthalmol Vis Sci 1991;32:2816–2820
109. Nikkinen A, Lehtosalo JI, Uusitalo H, et al. The lacrimal glands of the rat and guinea pig are innervated by nerve fibers containing immunoreactivities for substance P and vasoactive intestinal polypeptide. Histochemistry 1984;81:23–27
110. Matsumoto Y, Tanabe T, Ueda S, Kawata M. Immunohistochemical and enzyme histochemical studies of peptidergic, aminergic, and cholinergic innervation of the lacrimal gland of the monkey (*Macaca fuscata*). J Auton Nerv Syst 1992;37:207–214
111. Gibbins IL. Target-related patterns of co-existence of neuropeptide Y, vasoactive intestinal peptide, enkephalin, and substance P in cranial parasympathetic neurons innervating the facial skin and exocrine glands of guinea pigs. Neuroscience 1990;38:541–560
112. Maves CA, Rismondo V, Mircheff AK. Chronic stimulation of rabbit lacrimal acinar cells decreases intracellular pools of Na,K-ATPase and other surface enzymes. Invest Ophthalmol Vis Sci 1992;33s:1289

Hormonal Influences on the Lacrimal Gland

▬▬▬ Dwight W. Warren, Ph.D.

The lacrimal glands produce the major component of the aqueous tear film. Dry eyes resulting from lacrimal insufficiency are a major cause of ocular morbidity. The reasons for reduced lacrimal gland secretion can range from decreases in cellular function of the gland to Sjögren's syndrome, wherein this organ can be completely destroyed via an autoimmune process. Recent reviews of the literature show a marked, gender-related difference in the occurrence of lacrimal insufficiency [1]. Lacrimal insufficiency occurs especially frequently during pregnancy, oral contraceptive use, and after menopause, suggesting that hormonal factors play an important role in regulating lacrimal gland function [1, 2]. Sjögren's syndrome occurs ten times more frequently in women (predominantly postmenopausal women) than men [3], indicating a sexual dimorphism in lacrimal gland function as well as implicating hormonal factors in the progression of this autoimmune disease.

A number of investigators have noted that the lacrimal glands of male and female rats differ with respect to several morphological, biochemical, and functional parameters. In lacrimal glands of mature female rats, acini tend to be smaller [4–7] and to produce less secretory component [8]. Female lacrimal glands contain fewer IgA-positive B cells and plasmacytes [9] and secrete less IgA [10]. In at least one species, female lacrimal glands express significantly smaller numbers of beta-adrenergic receptors [11]. In contrast, lacrimal glands of female rats contain leucine aminopeptidase, which is virtually undetectable in male animals [12].

Analysis of the literature reveals a striking conundrum: Dry eye occurs predominantly in postmenopausal women, in whom estrogen levels are greatly depressed, and in women who are pregnant or taking birth control pills, in whom estrogen and prolactin levels are elevated [1, 2]. My colleagues and I have hypothesized that a resolution to this discrepancy might be achieved if androgens rather than estrogens are considered the hormonal mediators of the lacrimal gland. With the decline of function of the ovary at menopause, androgens as well as estrogens decrease. During high-estrogen states, such as pregnancy or with use of estrogen-containing birth control pills, the liver is stimulated to produce sex hormone–binding globulin (SHBG), which binds circulating androgens and lowers the free or active fraction of this class of steroids. Thus, the active androgens are probably decreased in both high- and low-estrogen states. As will be discussed later, prolactin levels also play an important role in lacrimal gland function.

The secretion of fluid and electrolytes involves multiple individual signal transduction and transport processes. Despite the large number of sexual dimorphisms described thus far, the literature contains virtually no information about possible gender-related differences in the lacrimal gland's ability to secrete electrolytes and water, and there are very few suggestions as to why women are more susceptible to lacrimal insufficiency. Recent work has identified key roles for Cl^- channels, K^+ channels, Na^+/H^+ and Cl^-/HCO_3^- antiporters, and Na^+,K^+-ATPase pumps [13]. The activities of these transporters are acutely regulated by the autonomic nervous system [14, 15]. Gender-dependent differences in the level of any of the transport proteins or secretomotor neurotransmitter receptors would be expected to influence lacrimal secretory function.

Current studies undertaken by my coworkers and I have focused on testing our hypothesis that androgens and prolactin regulate the biochemical correlates of exocrine secretion in the lacrimal gland. This chapter describes our specific studies to test this hypothesis as well as other known effects of androgens and prolactin on exocrine secretion.

■ Role of Androgens

Early studies demonstrated that castration of male rats decreases the size of lacrimal cells and that treatment with testosterone restores these cells to their larger, malelike appearance [6]. More recent studies by Sullivan and coworkers [8, 10, 16] have demonstrated that androgens play a major role in regulating the secretory immune system of the rat exorbital lacrimal gland. Interestingly, however, this same group has demonstrated that androgens fail to reverse the suppressive effects of hypophysectomy on the secretory immune system of the rat exorbital lacrimal gland [17, 18].

Recent studies on the development of lacrimal gland function in the rabbit have demonstrated that although lacrimal glands from prepubertal rabbits of either sex are remarkably similar, adult rabbits show distinct sexually dimorphic patterns with respect to correlates of secretion [19]. The lacrimal glands of male rabbits were nearly 30% larger and contained 45% more cells (as measured by total DNA) than lacrimal glands of female rabbits [19]. Additionally, beta-adrenergic receptors are increased by nearly 80% in male animals when compared to females [19]. Thus, there is a strong implication that androgens are responsible for increased levels of parameters correlated with secretory function in the rabbit lacrimal glands.

In more recent studies (DW Warren, AM Azzarolo, K Bjerrum, and AK Mircheff, unpublished data), the role of androgens on correlates of secretory function of the lacrimal gland in hypophysectomized female rats was assessed. Five days after hypophysectomy, the rats were treated for 2 days with dihydrotestosterone (DHT), a potent metabolite of testosterone that, unlike testosterone, is unable to be converted to estrogens. Hypophysectomy resulted in an approximately 50% decrease in almost all parameters measured. The effects of DHT were dramatic, increasing the total amount of DNA to approximately 50% above the levels in controls (animals that were not hypophysectomized). Total protein also was increased by DHT but not to the same extent as was seen for DNA. DHT partially increased the total amount of Na^+,K^+-ATPase as well as other membrane-bound enzymes (alkaline and acid phosphatases) and beta-adrenergic receptors. Interestingly, it had no effect on increasing muscarinic, cholinergic receptors (MAChRs), most likely the major transducer of neural stimulation–coupled lacrimal secretion. Thus, although androgens failed to reverse hypophysectomy-induced changes in the secretory immune system of the rat [17, 18], DHT was very potent in reversing, or at least partially ameliorating, the hypophysectomy-induced changes in exocrine secretory correlates of female rat lacrimal gland function.

The ovaries contribute approximately one-half of the total concentration of circulating androgens in the female animal. Thus, oophorectomy is one method of partially reducing androgens. In another series of experiments, oophorectomized rabbits displayed decreases in DNA, total and membrane-bound protein, Na^+,K^+-ATPase, and beta-adrenergic receptors. Treatment for 10 days with DHT again increased the total amount of DNA to well above control levels, as well as partially reversing the changes in total and membrane-bound protein and the membrane-associated enzymes and neurotransmitter receptors (DW Warren, AM Azzarolo, RL Kaswan, and AK Mircheff, unpublished data).

The hypothesis that it is low free androgen levels in both high- and low-estrogen states that affects lacrimal secretory function was tested by treating rabbits with high doses of the synthetic estrogen diethylstilbestrol (DES). Previous studies we conducted in the hypophysectomized rat model failed to demonstrate any effect of DES on lacrimal gland function. This observation is consistent with the data presented by Cornell-Bell and colleagues [4], who were unable to demonstrate the existence of any estrogen receptors in the lacrimal gland. Thus, treatment of rabbits with DES should increase SHBG and lower free androgens, resulting in depressed lacrimal gland function without directly affecting the lacrimal gland. Treatment of rabbits for 5 days with DES caused decreases in protein, DNA, and alkaline and acid phosphatase, changes consistent with the hypothesis that decreased androgens result in lowered levels of biochemical correlates of lacrimal gland secretion. The preceding data support the contention that androgens are one important component in maintaining lacrimal gland function.

■ Role of Prolactin

The studies of Sullivan and coworkers [8, 10, 16] demonstrating that hypophysectomized rats failed to respond to testosterone led to our investigation of possible pituitary hormone interaction with the lacrimal gland. Although any of the hormones from the pituitary gland might play a role in regulating lacrimal gland function, we chose to study the effects of prolactin because several reports in the literature implicate this hormone in lacrimal gland function. Frey and associates [20] demonstrated that prolactin-like immunoreactivity was present in human lacrimal gland and tears. Kaswan and colleagues [21, 22] demonstrated that cyclosporin A was useful in augmenting lacrimal secretion and may exert its action in lymphocytes by binding to prolactin receptors [23–25].

Our initial studies demonstrated receptors for prolactin along with immunohistochemical staining of prolactin in rat lacrimal gland acinar cells [26]. Whereas male rats appeared to have more receptors than female rats, this difference was not significant after endogenous prolactin was eluted from the receptors. Prolactin also inhibited acute carbachol-induced peroxidase release by lacrimal gland fragments, thus demonstrating a biological effect of prolactin. Additionally, prolactin mRNA was detected in male rat lacrimal glands but not in glands obtained from female animals [26].

To determine the effects of prolactin in the whole animal, we utilized the same hypophysectomized rat model as described previously when testing for androgen activity in the lacrimal gland. Prolactin, unlike DHT, had no effect on lacrimal gland DNA content and very slight, but significant, effects on total protein. However, prolactin significantly stimulated Na^+,K^+-ATPase and alkaline phosphatase activity as well as the number of MAChR, bringing these values to between 70% and 90% of controls. When assessed separately, it is clear that both androgen and prolactin treatment can replace most of the correlates of secretory function lost by hypophysectomy.

■ Synergy Between Androgens and Prolactin

In the same hypophysectomized female rat model, we assessed the combined effects of androgens and prolactin. Interestingly, we found no evidence of additive actions of the two hormones in any of the parameters measured. However, we did find evidence that prolactin could inhibit the effects of DHT and vice versa. Because prolactin suppressed carbachol-stimulated peroxidase release from rat lacrimal gland fragments and also stimulated various parameters of lacrimal gland function in the hypophysectomized rat, we hypothesized that this hormone might exert a biphasic effect in that concentrations above an optimal level for stimulation were inhibitory but, when below this level, were inadequate to support complete function. We observed support for this hypothesis in the hypophysectomized rat model, in that high doses of prolactin inhibited DHT-stimulated Na^+,K^+-ATPase, whereas low levels of prolactin did not affect the stimulatory action of DHT. There is also evidence for a biphasic effect of prolactin in rat ventral prostate cells in culture, where lower doses of prolactin were stimulatory and higher doses inhibitory [27].

It is possible that androgens have a biphasic effect as well. Whereas high doses of prolactin stimulated MAChR content and DHT had no effect, the combination of the two hormones elicited a significantly lesser response than the prolactin alone, indicating an inhibitory effect of DHT on prolactin stimulation of MAChR.

Clearly, additional work will be required to establish whether optimal prolactin levels contribute to normal lacrimal gland function. Nonetheless, the observed interactions between DHT and prolactin suggest the general hypothesis that the balance between prolactin and free androgen levels influences the lacrimal gland's gender-typical characteristics.

■ Conclusion

All the studies cited earlier that have evaluated the effects of androgens on lacrimal gland function have demonstrated that androgens unquestionably play a key role in the maintenance of the lacrimal gland, and thus they support the hypothesis that minimal levels of androgens are essential for normal lacrimal secretory function. If this hypothesis ultimately is validated by further evidence, then a strategy for treating non-Sjögren's lacrimal insufficiency after menopause and during oral contraceptive use with low-dose androgen treatment may be available in the near future. Although work remains to be done to test our tentative explanations for the excessive incidence of lacrimal insufficiency among women, it is already appropriate to initiate attempts to learn whether androgens and prolactin influence other transport proteins such as the Na^+/H^+ and Cl^-/HCO_3^- antiporters and Cl^- channels that mediate lacrimal NaCl secretion, the other neurotransmitter and neuropeptide receptors that modulate lacrimal secretion, and the intracellular messenger cascades by which such signals are transduced. It is appropriate also to begin examining the cellular and molecular mechanisms by which androgens and prolactin exert the actions that we have documented.

The nature of the role that pituitary gland prolactin plays in maintaining the lacrimal gland's functional status will be a particularly challenging field for exploration, complicated by the fact that prolactin or prolactin-like peptides may also function as local mediators within the lacrimal gland. Prolactin-like immunoreactivity is present in acinar cells of the human [20] and rat [26]. Acinar cells from both male and female rats contain similar numbers of receptors for prolactin, and recycling traffic between the basal-lateral plasma membrane and the endocytic compartments provides a pathway by which receptor-bound prolactin might be internalized and packaged for secretion. However, lacrimal glands also possess the ability to transcribe the prolactin message and, presumably, to synthesize prolactin [26]. Of particular interest is the fact that prolactin mRNA is detectable in lacrimal glands of male but not female rats. This suggests that lacrimal production of prolactin increases as circulating prolactin levels decrease, as the blood levels of prolactin are much lower in male than in female animals. The physiological implications of local prolactin production have yet to be investigated.

The author wishes to express his appreciation to the collaborators in the group who have made these studies possible: Drs. Austin K. Mircheff, Renee L. Kaswan, Richard L. Wood, and Kirsten Bjerrum, and Ms. Ana Maria Azzarolo, Ms. Barbara Platler, Ms. Diana Sayler, and Mr. Laren Becker.

These studies were supported in part by National Institutes of Health grant EY 09405, Bethesda, MD, and a University of Southern California School of Medicine Biomedical Research Support Grant from The National Institutes of Health to Dr. Warren, and National Institutes of Health grant EY 05801 to Dr. Mircheff.

■ References

1. Serrander A-M, Peek KE. Changes in contact lens comfort related to the menstrual cycle and menopause. A review of articles. J Am Optom Assoc 1993;64:162–166
2. Brennan NA, Effron N. Symptomatology of HEMA contact lens wear. Optom Vis Sci 1989;66:834–838
3. Molina R, Provost TT, Arnett FC, et al. Clinical serologic and immunogenetic features. Am J Med 1986;80:23–31
4. Cornell-Bell AH, Sullivan DA, Allansmith MR. Gender-related differences in the morphology of the lacrimal gland. Invest Ophthalmol Vis Sci 1985;26:1170–1175
5. Walker R. Age changes in the rat's exorbital lacrimal gland. Anat Rec 1958;132:49–69
6. Cavallero C. Relative effectiveness of various steroids in an androgen assay using the exorbital lacrimal gland of the castrated rat. Acta Endocrinol (Copenh) 1967;55:119–130
7. Hahn JD. Effect of cyproterone acetate on sexual dimorphism of the exorbital lacrimal gland in rats. J Endocrinol 1969;45:421–424
8. Sullivan DA, Bloch KJ, Allansmith MR. Hormonal influence on the secretory immune system of the eye: androgen regulation of secretory component levels in rat tears. J Immunol 1984;132:1130–1135

9. Hann LE, Allansmith MR, Sullivan DA. Impact of aging and gender on the Ig-containing cell profile of the lacrimal gland. Acta Ophthalmol (Copenh) 1988;66: 87–92
10. Sullivan DA, Allansmith MR. Hormonal regulation of the secretory immune system in the eye: androgen modulation of IgA levels in tears of rats. J Immunol 1985;134: 2978–2982
11. Pangerl A, Pangerl B, Jones DJ, Reiter RJ. Beta-adrenoreceptors in the extraorbital lacrimal gland of the Syrian hamster. Characterization with [125I]-iodopindolol and evidence of sexual dimorphism. J Neural Transm 1989;77:153–162
12. Lauria A, Porcelli F. Leucine aminopeptidase (LAP) activity and sexual dimorphism in rat exorbital lacrimal gland. Basic Appl Histochem 1979;23:171–177
13. Mircheff AK. Lacrimal fluid and electrolyte secretion: a review. Curr Eye Res 1989; 8:607–617
14. Thaysen JH. The lacrimal gland. In: Andreoli TE, Hoffman JF, Fanestil DD, eds. Physiology of membrane disorders. New York: Plenum, 1978:415
15. Lambert RW, Maves CA, Mircheff AK. Carbachol-induced increase of Na^+/H^+ antiport and recruitment of Na^+,K^+-ATPase in rabbit lacrimal acini. Curr Eye Res 1993;12:539–551
16. Sullivan DA, Bloch KJ, Allansmith MR. Hormonal influence on the secretory immune system of the eye: androgen control of secretory component production by the rat exorbital gland. Immunology 1984;52:239–246
17. Sullivan DA, Allansmith MR. Hormonal influence on the secretory immune system of the eye: endocrine interactions in the control of IgA and secretory component levels in tears of rats. Immunology 1987;60:337–343
18. Sullivan DA, Allansmith MR. Hormonal modulation of tear volume in the rat. Exp Eye Res 1986;42:131–139
19. Azzarolo AM, Mazaheri AH, Mircheff AK, Warren DW. Sex-dependent parameters related to electrolyte, water and glycoprotein secretion in rabbit lacrimal glands. Curr Eye Res 1994:in press
20. Frey WH, Nelson JD, Frick ML, Elde RP. Prolactin immunoreactivity in human tears and lacrimal gland: possible implications for tear production. In: Holly FJ, ed. The preocular tear film in health, disease, and contact lens wear. Lubbock, TX: Dry Eye Institute, 1986:798–807
21. Kaswan RL, Salisbury M-A, Ward DA. Spontaneous canine keratoconjunctivitis sicca. A useful model for human keratoconjunctivitis sicca: treatment with cyclosporine eye drops. Arch Ophthalmol 1989;107:1210–1216
22. Kaswan RL, Salisbury MA, Mircheff AK, Gierow JP. Lacromimetic effects of cyclosporine. Invest Ophthalmol Vis Sci 1990;31(suppl):46
23. Russell DH, Matrisian L, Kibler R, et al. Prolactin receptors on human lymphocytes and their modulation by cyclosporine. Biochem Biophys Res Commun 1984;121: 899–906
24. Larson DF. Mechanisms of action: antagonism of the prolactin receptor. Prog Allergy 1986;38:222–238
25. Hiestand PC, Mekler P, Nordmann R, et al. Prolactin as a modulator of lymphocyte responsiveness provides a possible mechanism of action for cyclosporine. Proc Natl Acad Sci USA 1986;83:2599–2603
26. Mircheff AK, Warren DW, Wood RL, et al. Prolactin localization, binding and effects on peroxidase release in rat exorbital lacrimal gland. Invest Ophthalmol Vis Sci 1992;33:641–650
27. Romero L, Munoz C, Lopez A, Vilches J. Effects of prolactin on explant cultures of rat ventral prostate: morphological and immunohistochemical study. Prostate 1993;22:1–10

Human Tear Film Electrolyte Concentrations in Health and Dry-Eye Disease

Jeffrey P. Gilbard, M.D.

Tear film osmolarity may be increased by any disorder that increases tear evaporation or decreases tear secretion, including meibomian gland dysfunction, due to chronic meibomianitis, and lacrimal gland disease, usually due to an autoimmune mechanism [1]. In both cases, the surface disease that results is known as *keratoconjunctivitis sicca* (KCS) and is characterized by decreased conjunctival goblet-cell density and corneal glycogen levels, characteristic epithelial abnormalities, and rose bengal staining [2–9].

For many years, investigators could not demonstrate elevated tear film osmolarity in KCS because of limitations in the techniques used to collect and study tear fluid [10]. These techniques required the collection of large volumes of tear fluid that, in turn, necessitated ocular contact and stimulation of tear secretion. Because tear film osmolarity decreases with increased flow rate, investigators documented increased osmolarity only after a technique was developed to collect and study tear samples as small as 0.1 µl [11–13].

Many studies in the literature report the results of human tear electrolyte measurements [14, 15]. Like the early tear osmolarity studies, these studies required relatively long collection times and stimulation of tear secretion to collect samples of adequate size. Because tear electrolyte concentrations change with lacrimal gland secretion rate [16], these studies were limited in their ability to measure electrolyte concentrations accurately in the normal and diseased tear film. Long collection times create an additional problem with regard to the measurement of bicarbonate as disassociated CO_2 gas can rapidly escape into adjacent air, reducing the amount of bicarbonate in the sample.

With the increasing recognition of the importance of tear electrolytes in maintaining the ocular surface [17–20], there has been increased interest in the electrolyte composition of the normal undisturbed tear film. I now report my clinical method for differentiating patients with meibomian gland dysfunction from those with lacrimal gland disease, as well as our findings regarding tear osmolarity and electrolyte measurements on microvolume tear samples collected from these patients and normal controls.

■ Patients and Methods

Patients with ocular irritation were divided prospectively into three groups based on history, examination, and rose bengal staining: (1) meibomian gland dysfunction (n = 9), (2) lacrimal gland disease (n = 19), and (3) lacrimal gland disease and meibomian gland dysfunction (n = 3).

Patients with meibomian gland dysfunction and patients with lacrimal gland disease both complained of a sandy-gritty irritation that worsened late in the day. In addition, patients with meibomian gland dysfunction frequently had a past or current history of a sandy-gritty irritation on awakening in the morning. These early-morning symptoms were attributed to meibomianitis. Some of the patients with lacrimal gland disease had a history of xerostomia or serologically documented Sjögren's syndrome.

The meibomian gland orifices normally are visible on the eyelid margin and, as such, are described as *open*. When a meibomian gland orifice is not visible on the eyelid margin but oil can be expressed by gentle lid pressure, the orifice is described as *stenosed*. If the orifice is not visible and oil cannot be expressed, it is termed *closed*. The status of the meibomian gland orifices for each eye was described using any combination of these terms (Fig 1).

Tear film volume was assessed by slit-lamp examination with and without fluorescein. Fluorescein is particularly helpful because it does not fluoresce well when tear volume is diminished. With relatively obvious decreases in tear volume, fluorescein remains dark throughout the entire tear film, whereas with small decreases only the nasal portion of the inferior marginal tear strip may fail to fluoresce. A wetted fluorescein strip

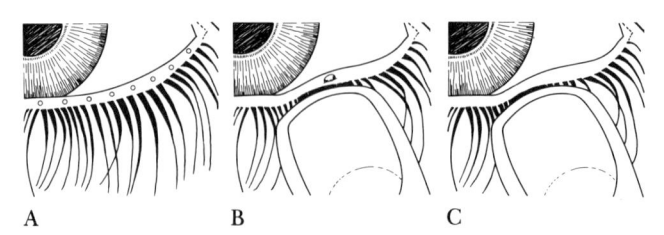

Figure 1 *Meibomian gland dysfunction grading system. (A) Patent meibomian gland orifices are visible on the eyelid margin. (B) Stenosed orifices are not visible, but oil can be expressed. (C) Closed orifices are not visible, and oil cannot be expressed.*

was touched briefly to the inferior tarsal conjunctiva and the tear film observed.

Patients assigned to the meibomian gland dysfunction group showed stenosis or closure of the meibomian gland orifices (or both) and had apparently normal tear volume; sometimes the tear film had a somewhat watery appearance, interpreted as loss of the normal lipid layer. Under McCulley's classification system for chronic blepharitis, these patients had primary meibomian keratoconjunctivitis in either the active or postinflammatory phase. This type of blepharitis commonly is associated with acne rosacea [21–23].

Patients assigned to the lacrimal gland disease group had patent meibomian gland orifices and a normal-appearing tear film, a tear film that appeared to have increased viscosity, or a tear film of diminished volume.

The rose bengal staining pattern was similar in all groups: limited to the bulbar conjunctiva within the exposure zones and, in the absence of meibomianitis, affecting the conjunctiva more than the cornea. For equivalent tear volumes, patients with meibomian gland dysfunction exhibited more rose bengal staining than those with lacrimal gland disease.

Patients assigned to the meibomian gland dysfunction–lacrimal gland disease group had stenosed or closed meibomian gland orifices and decreased tear film volume.

Samples for tear osmolarity and electrolyte measurement were obtained from a control group of 23 normal subjects (18 women and 5 men) and from 31 dry-eye patients (27 women and 4 men). Normal subjects denied eye symptoms, including dry-eye complaints, and had unremarkable examinations. Demographic data on the control and the dry-eye groups is provided in Table 1.

Tear samples of approximately 0.1 µl were collected from the inferior marginal tear strip with special L-shaped micropipettes that entered the strip without globe or eyelid contact [11]. Samples were stored as previously described [13]. Tear film osmolarity and electrolyte concentrations were measured using microtechniques that permitted all measurements to be made from each single tear collection sample. Tear osmolarity measurements were performed by freezing-point depression using a Clifton Nanolitre Osmometer (Clifton Technical Physics, Hartford, NY) [12]. Tear sodium (Na^+), potassium (K^+), calcium (Ca^{++}), and magnesium (Mg^{++})

Table 1 *Age (Years) of Normal Controls and Dry-Eye Patients*

Subject Group	Mean ± SEM	Range
Normals	46.9 ± 3.0	26–80
Meibomian gland dysfunction (MGD)	52.1 ± 3.9	35–69
Lacrimal gland disease (LGD)	51.6 ± 3.6	23–80
MGD and LGD	70.3 ± 6.7	58–81

were measured by atomic absorption spectrophotometry (Smith Heiftje 22, Thermo Jarrell Ash, Franklin, MA), as previously described [24]. Tear bicarbonate (HCO_3^-) levels were determined using a picapnotherm (model GV-1, World Precision Instruments, New Haven, CT), as previously described [25, 26].

Unless otherwise stated, measurements are averaged across eyes such that each individual is expressed as a single measurement. All data are expressed as the mean plus or minus the standard error of the mean (SEM). Each disease group was compared to normal controls. The Wilcoxon nonparametric test was used to perform overall tests of significance between groups. In addition, an analysis of variance was performed using Dunnett's t test to establish pairwise comparisons between groups. A regression analysis was performed using the normal controls to adjust for age as an explanatory variable for osmolarity and all electrolyte measurements. All analyses were conducted both with and without adjusting for age differences between the diseased groups and the normal controls. The differences between groups with respect to the concentration of sodium relative to the other electrolytes was assessed using the ratio of each electrolyte to sodium in a one-way analysis of variance.

■ Results

In the 23 normal subjects, tear film osmolarity measured in milliosmoles per liter was 304.4 ± 0.3 and ranged between 299 and 309. Tear film electrolytes, measured in millimoles per liter, were as follows: Na^+, 133.2 ± 0.2; K^+, 24.0 ± 0.2; HCO_3^-, 32.8 ± 0.04; Ca^{++}, 0.80 ± 0.0006; and Mg^{++}, 0.61 ± 0.0006 (Table 2, Figs 2 through 7).

Table 3 displays the results of the linear regression analysis of osmolarity and each electrolyte with regard to age in the normal controls. Age was a significant explanatory variable for all parameters except K^+. The annual rate in Table 3 represents the expected increase with age. For example, a 50-year-old normal control would be expected to have a 0.931-mosm/L

Table 2 *Tear Osmolarity (mosm/L) and Electrolyte Concentrations (mmol/L) in Normal Controls and Dry-Eye Patients*

Parameter	Normals	MGD	LGD	MGD & LGD
Osmolarity	304.4 ± 0.3	311.5 ± 1.1	316.2 ± 0.9	317.2 ± 1.1
Sodium	133.2 ± 0.2	136.1 ± 0.5	142.2 ± 0.5	145.1 ± 0.5
Potassium	24.0 ± 0.2	24.6 ± 0.1	24.9 ± 0.1	25.4 ± 0.1
Bicarbonate	32.8 ± 0.04	33.6 ± 0.1	34.3 ± 0.1	34.6 ± 0.1
Calcium	0.80 ± 0.0006	0.82 ± 0.002	0.84 ± 0.003	0.86 ± 0.003
Magnesium	0.61 ± 0.0006	0.62 ± 0.002	0.63 ± 0.002	0.65 ± 0.002

MGD = meibomian gland dysfunction; LGD = lacrimal gland disease.

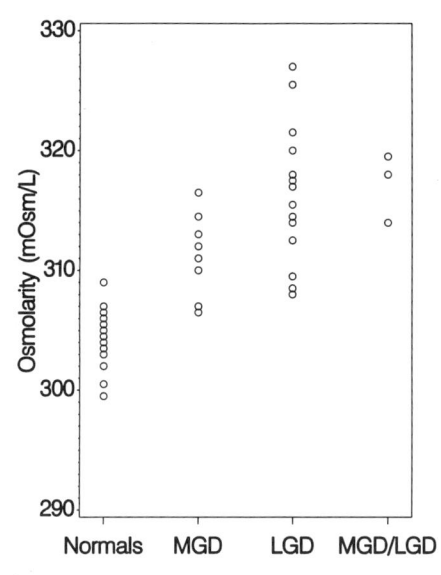

Figure 2 Tear film osmolarity averaged across eyes in normals and patients with meibomian gland dysfunction (MGD), lacrimal gland disease (LGD), and combined meibomian gland dysfunction and lacrimal gland disease (MGD/LGD).

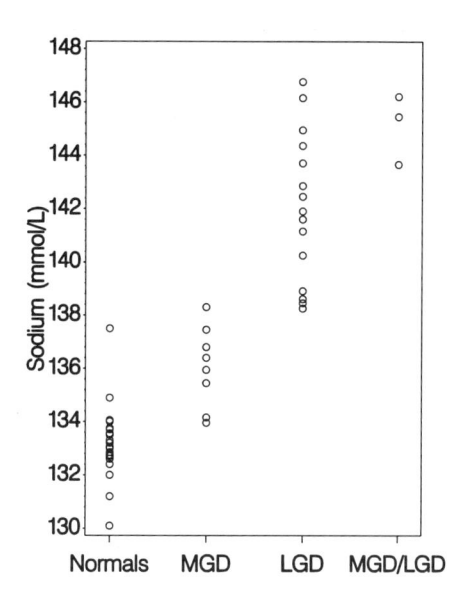

Figure 3 Tear film sodium averaged across eyes in normals and patients with meibomian gland dysfunction (MGD), lacrimal gland disease (LGD), and combined meibomian gland dysfunction and lacrimal gland disease (MGD/LGD).

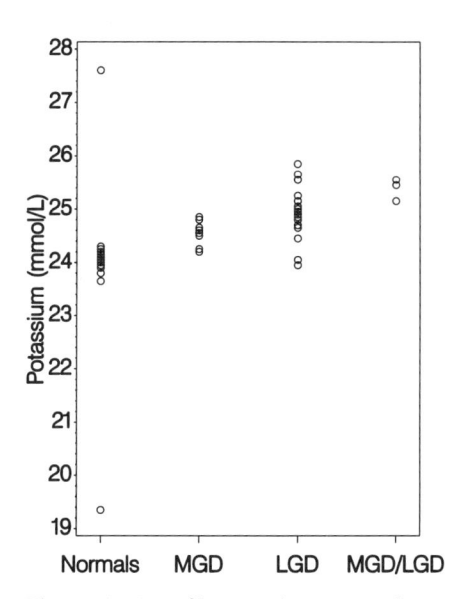

Figure 4 Tear film potassium averaged across eyes in normals and patients with meibomian gland dysfunction (MGD), lacrimal gland disease (LGD), and combined meibomian gland dysfunction and lacrimal gland disease (MGD/LGD).

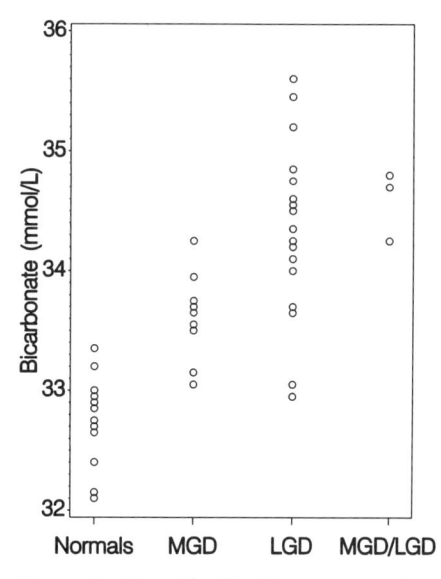

Figure 5 Tear film bicarbonate averaged across eyes in normals and patients with meibomian gland dysfunction (MGD), lacrimal gland disease (LGD), and combined meibomian gland dysfunction and lacrimal gland disease (MGD/LGD).

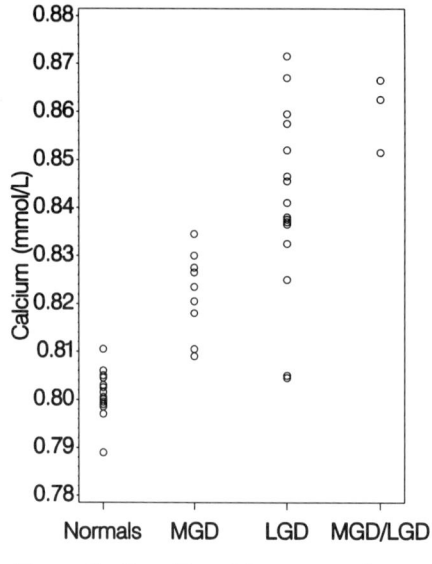

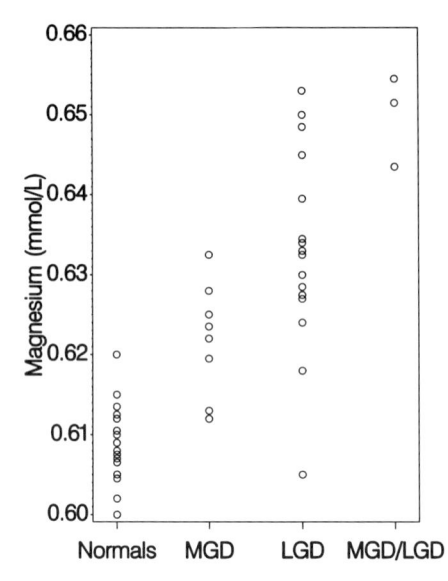

Figure 6 *Tear film calcium averaged across eyes in normals and patients with meibomian gland dysfunction* (MGD), *lacrimal gland disease* (LGD), *and combined meibomian gland dysfunction and lacrimal gland disease* (MGD/LGD).

Figure 7 *Tear film magnesium averaged across eyes in normals and patients with meibomian gland dysfunction* (MGD), *lacrimal gland disease* (LGD), *and combined meibomian gland dysfunction and lacrimal gland disease* (MGD/LGD).

increase in osmolarity (10 × 0.0931) relative to a 40-year-old normal control. Using the linear regression to adjust all normals to the age of 40, tear film osmolarity averages 303.7 mosm/L ± 0.4 and ranges between 300 and 307. Tear film electrolytes in millimoles per liter are as follows: Na^+, 132.8 ± 0.2; K^+, 23.8 ± 0.3; HCO_3^-, 32.7 ± 0.04; Ca^{++}, 0.80 ± 0.0007; and Mg^{++}, 0.61 ± 0.0008.

In the meibomian gland dysfunction group, mean tear osmolarity and tear Na^+, K^+, HCO_3^-, Ca^{++}, and Mg^{++} concentrations increased uniformly by approximately 2% (see Table 2 and Figs 2 through 7). Both with and without adjustment for age, all increases except that observed for K^+ were significant at the 0.05 level.

Table 3 *Effect of Age on Tear Film Osmolarity and Electrolyte Concentrations in 23 Normal Controls*

Parameter	Annual Rate	Annual Standard Error	*p* Value
Osmolarity	0.0931 mosm/L	0.0254	0.0015
Sodium	0.0561 mmol/L	0.0169	0.0032
Potassium	0.0289 mmol/L	0.0289	0.1288
Bicarbonate	0.0138 mmol/L	0.0031	0.0002
Calcium	0.00016 mmol/L	0.00005	0.0047
Magnesium	0.00017 mmol/L	0.00006	0.0067

There were 5 eyes from 4 patients in the meibomian gland dysfunction group that had tear osmolarity of less than 310 mosm/L. In these eyes, osmolarity was 305.6 ± 1.6 mosm/L; tear electrolytes in millimoles per liter measured as follows: Na$^+$, 133.6 ± 0.7; K$^+$, 24.1 ± 0.1; HCO$_3^-$, 33.0 ± 0.2; Ca^{++}, 0.81 ± 0.004; and Mg^{++}, 0.61 ± 0.003. Averaging across eyes and adjusting for age, these electrolyte concentrations were not significantly different from normal.

In the lacrimal gland disease group, tear film osmolarity and tear film K$^+$, HCO$_3^-$, Ca^{++}, and Mg^{++} increased by about 3.5% relative to controls. Tear film Na$^+$, however, increased disproportionately by 6.8% relative to controls (see Table 2 and Figs 2 through 7). Both with and without adjustment for age, all increases were significant at the 0.05 level. In addition, the Na$^+$ ratio analysis, adjusted for age, indicated that the disproportionate increase in Na$^+$ relative to all the remaining electrolytes was significant at the 0.05 level.

Among patients in the lacrimal gland disease group, there were 5 eyes with osmolarity measurements of less than 310 mosm/L. In these patients, osmolarity was 308.4 ± 0.4 mosm/L; tear electrolytes in millimoles per liter measured as follows: Na$^+$, 138.4 ± 0.2; K$^+$, 24.1 ± 0.1; HCO$_3^-$, 33.1 ± 0.2; Ca^{++}, 0.81 ± 0.004; and Mg^{++}, 0.61 ± 0.003. Averaging across eyes and adjusting for age, the 3.9% increase in Na$^+$ was significant at the 0.05 level; the remaining electrolyte concentrations were not significantly different from normal.

Patients in the meibomian gland dysfunction–lacrimal gland disease group retained the disproportionate increase in tear Na$^+$ (see Table 2). In addition, the increases in both tear osmolarity and tear electrolyte concentrations were highest in this group (see Table 2 and Figs 2 through 7). When not age-adjusted, the increases in osmolarity, Na$^+$, K$^+$, HCO$_3^-$, Ca^{++}, and Mg^{++} were all significant at the 0.05 level; when age-adjusted, the increase in K$^+$ was no longer significant. The Na$^+$ ratio analysis, adjusted for age, indicated that the disproportionate increase in Na$^+$, relative to all the remaining electrolytes except K$^+$, was significant at the 0.05 level.

■ Comments

Reported here for the first time are tear film electrolyte concentrations in unstimulated microvolume tear samples, collected rapidly without conjunctival trauma, from both normal subjects and patients with the most commonly encountered varieties of dry-eye disease. The differing tear electrolyte profiles observed in patients with a clinical diagnosis of meibomian gland or lacrimal gland disease confirm the validity of the diagnostic approach outlined in this study. Based on history, examination, and rose bengal staining, and independent of Schirmer testing, it is possible to separate patients with dry-eye symptoms into those with disease resulting from meibomian gland dysfunction and those with disease resulting from lacrimal gland disease.

In previous work with rabbit models, my colleagues and I found that meibomian gland dysfunction alone is sufficient to increase tear film osmolarity [7]. The current clinical data provide additional evidence that meibomian gland dysfunction, independent of any lacrimal gland disease, can increase tear film osmolarity and produce dry-eye disease.

Meibomian gland dysfunction increases tear electrolytes uniformly and in proportion with tear osmolarity, consistent with a purely evaporative effect. In contrast, while lacrimal gland disease increases osmolarity and tear K^+ and HCO_3^- uniformly consistent with an evaporative effect, there is a disproportionate increase in tear Na^+. This disproportionate increase in tear Na^+ is consistent with increased Na^+ in the primary lacrimal gland secretion at the low flow rates observed in lacrimal gland disease.

Botelho and Martinez [16] studied tear Na^+, K^+, and chloride concentrations in fluid collected directly from the rabbit lacrimal gland excretory duct at various flow rates. They found that at low flow rates, Na^+ and chloride concentrations increased, independent of the effects of evaporation. In contrast, tear K^+ levels remained unchanged at moderate and low flow rates (all flow rates less than 2 μl/min). The increase in tear Na^+ observed in patients with very early lacrimal gland disease and normal tear osmolarity, and the disproportionate increase in tear Na^+ seen in patients with lacrimal gland disease and elevated tear osmolarity, are most likely due to the phenomenon originally described by Botelho and Martinez.

We recently demonstrated in the rabbit that lacrimal gland fluid osmolarity increases as flow rate declines, independent of the effects of evaporation [27]. The disproportionate increases in tear Na^+ in patients with lacrimal gland disease makes it likely that tear osmolarity increases in these patients in part due to higher lacrimal gland fluid osmolarity at low flow rates. This increase in lacrimal gland fluid osmolarity at low flow rates is a result of increased lacrimal gland fluid Na^+.

Elevated tear film osmolarity was not an entry criteria for the dry-eye patient groups, which enabled us to study changes in tear electrolyte concentrations that may precede increases in tear film osmolarity. It is noteworthy that there were 5 eyes in which the diagnosis was lacrimal gland disease that had normal tear osmolarity but elevated tear Na^+. This suggests that increased tear Na^+ precedes increased tear osmolarity in early lacrimal gland disease. It may be that initial associated increases in lacrimal gland fluid osmolarity are obscured in the tear film by the osmotically driven transport of water across the cornea and conjunctiva [28]. Such osmotically driven water transport can normalize tear osmolarity but not tear Na^+. In early KCS, ocular surface disease may be due to changes in the secreted lacrimal gland fluid, as opposed to an increase in the influence of tear film evaporation secondary to decreased tear film turnover or decreased volume. This data also suggests that tear volume is not necessarily decreased in early KCS.

In the group of normal subjects, age was a significant explanatory variable for osmolarity and all electrolytes measured except K^+. The effect of age was most significant for Na^+ and HCO_3^-. The age-adjusted ratio of Na^+ to HCO_3^- in the tear film of normal subjects (132.8/32.7 = 4.061) was equivalent to the ratio of the annual change in Na^+ with age to the annual change in HCO_3^- with age (0.0561/0.0138 = 4.0652). This indicates that the gradual linear increase in tear film osmolarity observed with age was not associated with a disproportionate increase in tear Na^+. It suggests that the increase in osmolarity and electrolyte concentrations seen in normals with age is secondary to a gradual increase in tear film evaporation rather than a decrease in tear secretion. This putative increase in tear film evaporation is probably attributable to a normal gradual decline in meibomian gland function with increasing age.

We previously found that conjunctival goblet-cell density is sensitive to changes in the electrolyte composition of bathing solutions [19, 20]. Our investigations revealed an optimum electrolyte balance for maintaining conjunctival goblet cells that matches the electrolyte balance we now report in the normal human tear film. It also is significant that with lacrimal gland disease, tear Na^+ increases to more than 140 mmol/L, a level that is incompatible with the maintenance of normal conjunctival goblet-cell density [19, 20]. We now hypothesize that disproportionate increases in tear Na^+, along with increases in tear osmolarity, may contribute to the development of surface disease, specifically the loss of conjunctival goblet cells, in patients with lacrimal gland disease.

This work was presented in part at a meeting of the Association for Research in Vision and Ophthalmology, Sarasota, FL, May 3–8, 1992. It was supported in part by grant EY03373 from the National Eye Institute, Bethesda, MD, and by the Massachusetts Lions Eye Research Fund, Inc.

Scott R. Rossi, M.S., provided technical assistance. Philip T. Lavin, Ph.D., performed the statistical analysis.

An electrolyte-based ophthalmic solution invented by the author has been issued U.S. patents 4,775,531 and 4,911,933, and Canadian patent 1,263,606. Additional foreign patents have been issued or are pending. The Schepens Eye Research Institute is the assignee. The institute and the author have a proprietary interest in this technology.

■ References

1. Gilbard JP, Rossi SR, Gray KL. Mechanisms for increased tear film osmolarity. In: Cavanagh HD, ed. The cornea: transactions of the World Congress on the Cornea III. New York: Raven Press, 1988:5–7
2. Ralph RA. Conjunctival goblet cell density in normal subjects and in dry eye syndromes. Invest Ophthalmol Vis Sci 1975;14:299–302
3. Nelson JD, Havener VR, Cameron JD. Cellulose acetate impressions of the ocular surface. Dry eye states. Arch Ophthalmol 1983;101:1869–1872
4. Nelson JD, Wright JC. Conjunctival goblet cell densities in ocular surface disease. Arch Ophthalmol 1984;102:1049–1051

5. Abdel-Khalek LMR, Williamson J, Lee WR. Morphological changes in the human conjunctival epithelium. II. In keratoconjunctivitis sicca. Br J Ophthalmol 1978;62: 800–806
6. Gilbard JP, Rossi S, Gray K. A new rabbit model for keratoconjunctivitis sicca. Invest Ophthalmol Vis Sci 1987;28:225–228
7. Gilbard JP, Rossi SR, Gray Heyda K. Tear film and ocular surface changes after closure of the meibomian gland orifices in the rabbit. Ophthalmology 1989;96: 1180–1186
8. Gilbard JP, Rossi SR, Gray KL, et al. Tear film osmolarity and ocular surface disease in two rabbit models for keratoconjunctivitis sicca. Invest Ophthalmol Vis Sci 1988; 29:374–378
9. Gilbard JP, Rossi SR, Gray KL, Hanninen LA. Natural history of disease in a rabbit model for keratoconjunctivitis sicca. Acta Ophthalmol (Copenh) 1989;(suppl 192)67:95–101
10. Mastman GJ, Baldes EJ, Henderson JW. The total osmotic pressure of tears in normal and various pathologic conditions. Arch Ophthalmol 1961;65:509–513
11. Gilbard JP, Farris RL, Santamaria J. Osmolarity of tear microvolumes in keratoconjunctivitis sicca. Arch Ophthalmol 1978;96:677–681
12. Gilbard JP, Farris RL. Ocular surface drying and tear film osmolarity in thyroid eye disease. Acta Ophthalmol (Copenh) 1983;61:108–116
13. Gilbard JP, Gray KL, Rossi SR. Improved technique for storage of tear microvolumes. Invest Ophthalmol Vis Sci 1987;28:401–403
14. Van Haeringen NJ. Clinical biochemistry of tears. Surv Ophthalmol 1981;26:84–96
15. Rismondo V, Osgood TB, Leering P, et al. Electrolyte composition of lacrimal gland fluid and tears of normal and vitamin A deficient rabbits. CLAO J 1989;15:222–229
16. Botelho SY, Martinez EV. Electrolytes in lacrimal gland fluid and in tears at various flow rates in the rabbit. Am J Physiol 1973;225:606–609
17. Bachman WG, Wilson G. Essential ions for maintenance of the corneal epithelial surface. Invest Ophthalmol Vis Sci 1985;26:1484–1488
18. Fullard RJ, Wilson GS. Investigation of sloughed corneal epithelial cells collected by non-invasive irrigation of the corneal surface. Curr Eye Res 1986;5:847–856
19. Gilbard JP. Non-toxic ophthalmic preparations: US Patent 4,775,531. Oct 4, 1988
20. Gilbard JP, Rossi SR, Gray Heyda K. Ophthalmic solutions, the ocular surface, and a unique therapeutic artificial tear formulation. Am J Ophthalmol 1989;107:348–355
21. McCulley JP. Blepharoconjunctivitis. Int Ophthalmol Clin 1984;24:65–77
22. McCulley JP, Dougherty JM. Blepharitis associated with acne rosacea and seborrheic dermatitis. Int Ophthalmol Clin 1985;25:159–172
23. Bowman RW, Miller KN, McCulley JP. Diagnosis and treatment of chronic blepharitis. In: Wagner MD, ed. Focal points 1989, vol 7, mod 10: clinical modules for ophthalmologists. San Francisco: American Academy of Ophthalmology, 1989
24. Gilbard JP, Rossi SR. Tear film and ocular surface changes in a rabbit model of neurotrophic keratitis. Ophthalmology 1990;97:308–312
25. Vurek GG, Warnock DG, Corsey R. Measurement of picomole amounts of carbon dioxide by calorimetry. Anal Chem 1975;47:765–767
26. Bowman RL, Vurek GG. Analysis of nanoliter biological samples. Anal Chem 1984; 56:391A–405A
27. Gilbard JP, Dartt DA. Changes in rabbit lacrimal gland fluid osmolarity with flow rate. Invest Ophthalmol Vis Sci 1982;23:804–806
28. Maurice D. The tonicity of an eye drop and its dilution by tears. Exp Eye Res 1971;11:30–33

Diagnosis of Keratoconjunctivitis Sicca

J. Daniel Nelson, M.D., F.A.C.S.

It is difficult to define the term *dry eye,* as there are numerous causes of dry eye, many of which are not tied to lack of tear production. Compounding the difficulty is the fact that *dry eye* is defined differently by patient and ophthalmologist. For the patient, a dry eye is identified by subjective feelings—a foreign-body sensation, burning, and dryness, whereas the ophthalmologist usually identifies the condition using the Schirmer test. The terms *dry eye* and *keratoconjunctivitis sicca* (KCS) often are equated, but it probably is best to separate these terms. For this discussion, *dry eye* will be used to refer to a group of diseases characterized by patient symptoms due to an abnormal tear film and ocular surface. KCS will be defined as a specific type of dry-eye condition, characterized by a qualitative or quantitative abnormality of lacrimal gland secretion that results in an abnormal tear film and ocular surface. Note that the terms *tear film* and *ocular surface* are used together; this is because a normal ocular surface depends on a normal tear film and vice versa.

The cause of the patient's dry eye must be determined. Armed with a specific diagnosis, the ophthalmologist can recommend specific therapeutic interventions, the importance of which cannot be overemphasized. A specific diagnosis allows determination of how aggressively one should approach therapy. Patient compliance is virtually ensured when specific therapies are employed because symptoms improve. In addition, potential toxic therapies and side effects of unnecessary or ineffective medications are avoided.

Several causes of dry eye may be present in the same patient. For instance, blepharitis and KCS often are found together, and both must be treated to resolve patient symptoms.

■ Causes of KCS

KCS, the lack of sufficient quality or quantity of lacrimal gland secretions to maintain the tear film and ocular surface, is usually due to abnormalities of stimulation of tear secretion, destruction of the lacrimal and accessory lacrimal glands, or scarring or occlusion of the lacrimal gland secretory ducts. The most severe forms of KCS are due to destruction or absence of the lacrimal gland and include Sjögren's syndrome, the acquired immunodeficiency syndrome (AIDS) [1], graft-versus-host disease (GVHD) [2], and congenital and surgical removal of the lacrimal gland. Less severe forms of KCS occur due to abnormalities of the regulation of tear secretion, such as are brought on by aging, alterations in hormone levels (menopause), and systemic medications. Ocular surface diseases, such as ocular cicatricial pemphigoid, lichen planus, Stevens-Johnson syndrome, chemical burns, and GVHD, can cause KCS through the scarring, narrowing, and obliteration of the lacrimal and accessory lacrimal gland secretory ducts.

Blepharospasm and dermatochalasis are two great mimickers of KCS that often are missed on examination. Both diseases present with dry-eye symptoms and minimal findings of KCS. In the case of blepharospasm, there is spontaneous, nonvoluntary eyelid closure that results in symptoms. In dermatochalasis, the excessive weight of the upper eyelid skin causes the patient to elevate the brow, thereby instigating a decreased blink rate, increased evaporation, and poor spreading of the tear film [3]. The chronic brow elevation causes fatigue; its effects cause dry eye.

Blepharitis, allergy, and toxic keratoconjunctivitis magnify KCS. In patients with blepharitis, abnormalities of meibomian gland secretion lead to disruption of the lipid layer, resultant tear film instability, and increased evaporation [4]. The lack of aqueous tear secretion may predispose to blepharitis as a consequence of increased levels of bacterial flora resulting from decreased levels of tear IgA, lactoferrin, and lysozyme. KCS is more common in patients with rosacea [5]. In KCS, the lack of tears results in an inability to dilute or wash out allergens, increasing the likelihood of allergic conjunctivitis. Inflammatory products released by the allergic response, as well as eye rubbing, can worsen clinical symptoms and findings. The lack of aqueous tear secretion in KCS also results in an inability to dilute or wash out substances that may be placed in the eye, either purposely in the form of topical lubricants or medications or inadvertently by the application of cosmetics to the face and eyelids. Preservatives disrupt the lipid layer, leading to increased evaporation and tear film instability. In addition, preservatives, especially benzalkonium chloride, and many topical medications such as antibiotics are toxic to the epithelium [6–8]. Inability to dilute or wash out potentially toxic substances can cause epithelial and tear film abnormalities.

■ History

To determine whether a patient has KCS or some other cause of a dry eye, a careful, thorough history and clinical examination must be performed, supplemented by clinical and laboratory tests, tissue biopsy, and treatment trials.

It is curious that patients with acute external ocular disease will maximize their symptoms, whereas those with chronic disease tend to minimize symptoms. This may explain why some patients with severe discomfort have minimal clinical findings and some patients with significant clinical findings have rather minimal symptoms. Despite this, a careful history often will give the best clues to the proper diagnosis (Table 1). The character of the patient's pain or discomfort should be determined by both open-ended and specific questioning. Patients with KCS have particular, definable symptoms (Table 2), the most frequent being foreign-body sensation, burning, and photophobia. Patients often will use the term *dryness* to describe their condition but will have difficulty defining exactly what it means. Some will report a feeling of the eyelids grating or rubbing on the eye. The term *discomfort* may be a more accurate summation of all the patient's symptoms. Watery eyes or epiphora often is attributed to KCS, but other causes, such as blepharitis, dermatochalasis [3], and nasolacrimal duct obstruction, must be sought.

Symptoms should be rated or scored in some manner. A simple scale of absent (0), mild (1+), moderate (2+), and severe (3+) is useful. Let the patient rate the severity of his or her various symptoms and then use that rating at subsequent visits to assess improvement or worsening of symptoms.

Patients should be questioned as to whether they can produce irritant and emotional tears. Ask, "Do you get tears when you peel onions?" "Can you cry when you feel sad or hurt?" Affirmative responses suggest lacrimal glands in which some function remains, whereas negative answers suggest that the lacrimal gland is incapable of secreting tear fluid in response to any stimuli. In patients with KCS, the ability to generate irritant tears is lost before the ability to generate emotional tears.

The time course of these symptoms is important. How long have these symptoms been present? Are they related to the menstrual cycle, menopause, or hysterectomy or oophorectomy? Are there hour-to-hour, day-to-day, or month-to-month fluctuations? In patients with KCS, symptoms are usually less pronounced on awakening and worsen as the day progresses. Patients with blepharitis are highly symptomatic on awakening, better within an hour or so, and worse again later in the day. Are symptoms worsening as the patient ages? Is there a seasonal component? What effect does the patient's environment have on his or her symptoms? Patients with KCS are worse in dry, cold environments and under conditions of increased evaporation. Air drafts from air conditioners, car heaters, and ovens worsen symptoms. Determining whether symptoms are worse or better inside or out, at work or at home, will aid in identifying environments that need to be modified to improve patient symptoms.

Ask the patient what is being done now and what has been done in the past to treat the dry-eye condition. A detailed list of any topical lubri-

Table 1 Comparison of Historical Findings in Patients with Different Dry-Eye Disorders

Symptom	KCS	Blepharitis	Toxic KC	Allergic KC
Foreign-body sensation	+++	+	+++	+
Burning	+	+++	+++	+
Itching	−	−	−	+++
Photophobia	++	±	++	±
Crusting or mattering of lids	±	++	±	±
Symptoms worse	Afternoon, evening	On awakening	When using eye drops	Seasonal, environmental
Symptoms better	On awakening, morning	Midday	When not using drops	Different environment
Mucous discharge	++	+++	±	+++
Effect of preserved artificial tears on symptoms and signs	Worsens	±	Worsens	−
Effect of nonpreserved artificial tears on symptoms and signs	Improves	Improves	Worsens	Improves
Systemic anticholinergics	Symptoms worsen	±	±	
Systemic antihistamines	Symptoms worsen	±	±	Symptoms improve
Systemic disease	Collagen vascular disease, Sjögren's syndrome	Rosacea, seborrheic dermatitis	None	Atopic dermatitis, hay fever

KCS = keratoconjunctivitis sicca; KC = keratoconjunctivitis.
Source: Reprinted with permission from JD Nelson, Dry eye syndromes. In AP Schachat (ed), Current practice in ophthalmology. St Louis, MO: Mosby Year Book, 1992:54.
+ = present (additional + with increased severity)
− = absent
± = may be present

Table 2 *Definition of Patient Symptoms in Keratoconjunctivitis Sicca*

Symptom	Description
Foreign-body sensation	Feeling of sand or gravel in eyes
Burning	Feeling of soap or shampoo in the eyes
Photophobia	Discomfort on exposure to light
Itching	Sensation similar to a mosquito bite

cants and medications must be obtained, including drops as well as ointments. Inquire about these specifically, as most patients will not consider topical treatments when asked generally about medications. Are the topical lubricants preserved or unpreserved? How long have they been used and how often? Do they help (i.e., do they improve patient symptoms) and, if so, for how long? Most patients with KCS improve with topical lubricant therapy. Be wary of making the diagnosis of KCS if topical lubricants do not help at least somewhat. The severity of the patient's KCS often can be determined by how frequently topical lubricants are used: Patients with severe KCS use topical lubricants more often than those with mild KCS. Remember that patients with moderate to severe KCS often are made worse by topical lubricants containing preservatives (Table 3). Furthermore, any topical medication is potentially toxic due to the patient's inability to dilute it because of a lack of aqueous tear secretion.

Patients should be asked whether they have had previous placement of temporary collagen plugs. If so, note whether there was improvement in symptoms and whether epiphora occurred (and, if so, for how long). Ask if and when silicone punctal plugs were placed or whether previous permanent occlusion with laser or cautery has been performed. If punctal occlusion was done, did symptoms improve or, at least, did it allow a decrease in the use of topical lubricants?

The use of systemic medications must also be noted, as many systemic medications affect tear secretion (Table 4). Systemic antihistamines, antide-

Table 3 *Common Topical Lubricants and Their Preservatives*

Artificial Lubricants	Manufacturer	Preservative
Hypotears	IOLAB	Benzalkonium chloride
Tears Naturale	Alcon	Benzalkonium chloride
Tears Naturale II	Alcon	Polyquad
Liquifilm	Allergan	Chlorobutanol
Tears Plus	Allergan	Chlorobutanol
Moisture Drops	Bausch and Lomb	Benzalkonium chloride
Murine	Ross	Benzalkonium chloride
Tears Renewed	Akorn	Benzalkonium chloride
Akwa Tears	Akorn	Benzalkonium chloride

Table 4 *Systemic Medications That May Decrease Lacrimal Gland Secretion*

Medication Class	Type of Medication
Antihistamines	Hay fever and sleep medications
Antihypertensives	Beta-blockers, diuretics, methyldopa
Antiparkinsonian agents	Anticholinergics (e.g., Cogentin)
Antitussives	Opiates, anticholinergics
Belladonna alkaloids	Atropine, scopolamine
Psychotropics	Benzodiazepines, monoamine oxidase inhibitors, phenothiazines, tricyclic antidepressants

pressants, anticholinergics, and diuretics are most responsible for decreased lacrimal gland secretion. The use of systemic steroids and other immunosuppressives, such as hydroxychloroquine (Plaquenil), methotrexate, and cyclophosphamide (Cytoxan), which may be used in treating patients with Sjögren's syndrome and other collagen vascular diseases, should be noted. Patients with decreased tear secretion are at risk for ocular surface infections owing to decreased levels of tear immunoglobulins, lactoferrin, and lysozyme. The use of systemic immunosuppressives puts the patient at even greater risk.

It is important to determine whether the patient has any associated systemic symptoms or diseases. Therefore, a careful review of organ systems is required (Table 5). Important questions should be directed toward detecting a history of dry mouth (xerostomia) or dental and gum disease. Patients with Sjögren's syndrome and xerostomia are at increased risk of dental and gum disease owing to lack of saliva. Questions that help in determining whether the patient has significant xerostomia include the

Table 5 *Systemic Symptoms That May Be Associated with Dry Eyes*

Organ System	Disease or Symptoms
Ears, nose, throat	Nasal dryness, recurrent otitis media, parotid gland enlargement, xerostomia, caries, gum disease
Respiratory	Recurrent bronchitis, pneumonia
Genitourinary	Frequent bladder infections, decreased vaginal secretions
Gastrointestinal	Constipation, achlorhydria
Endocrine	Hypothyroidism, Graves' disease (exophthalmos, decreased blinking)
Dermatological	Seborrhea, rosacea, atopic dermatitis
Musculoskeletal	Joint pain and inflammation, Raynaud's phenomena
Neurological	Parkinson's disease (decreased blinking), Bell's palsy (lagophthalmos), multiple sclerosis
Skin	Dryness, petechial rash, eczema, rosacea
Other	Fatigue

following: Can you feel saliva in your mouth? Can you swallow bread or meat without additional fluids? Women should be asked whether they have experienced a noticeable decrease in vaginal secretions. Patients should be questioned about whether they have ever been told they have Sjögren's syndrome, systemic lupus erythematosus (SLE), rheumatoid arthritis (RA), systemic sclerosis (scleroderma), vasculitis, thyroid disease, lymphoma, or AIDS. If the patient has had a bone marrow transplant, find out whether he or she has suffered GVHD or rejection. Many patients with Sjögren's syndrome have significant fatigue, necessitating afternoon naps. A family history should be obtained, specifically asking whether there is a blood relative with KCS, Sjögren's syndrome, collagen vascular disease, and other eye diseases.

■ Clinical Examination

Nonocular Examinations

Before the eyes are examined, a limited physical examination is required. The facial skin is examined for evidence of acne rosacea and the malar rash of SLE. The scalp is examined for seborrheic dermatitis (dandruff). The parotid, submandibular, and submaxillary glands are palpated for the presence of enlargement or masses. Salivary gland enlargement is seen in patients with Sjögren's syndrome (formally called *Mikulicz's syndrome*); there is an increased risk of lymphomas in these patients. The thyroid gland is palpated for enlargement and nodules. Hypothyroidism is commonly seen in patients with Sjögren's syndrome, whereas hyperthyroidism is seen in some patients with Theodore's superior limbic keratoconjunctivitis (SLK). Exophthalmos and decreased blinking, which occur in Graves' disease, can cause symptoms and findings of dry eye due to increased evaporation. The mouth is examined for the presence or absence of saliva and for oral candidiasis, and the condition of the teeth and gums are noted. The tongue also is examined for evidence of dryness. The hands are assessed for joint inflammation and changes indicative of RA and scleroderma. Petechial rashes and eczema should be sought on the extremities.

Ocular Examinations

It is important to observe the patient's eyes and eyelids before proceeding with the slit-lamp examination. The severity of dermatochalasis, the palpebral fissure width, and the presence of brow wrinkling or elevation are noted. Patients with significant dermatochalasis often maintain a chin-up posture to improve their vision. Function of the eyelids, completeness of the blink, and the blink rate are assessed: Do the eyelids meet with each blink? Is ptosis present? Is there lagophthalmos with a normal blink, gentle, sleeplike closure, or forced eyelid closure?

The size of the lacrimal glands is evaluated by asking the patient to look down and out while the upper eyelid is retracted. Although it takes some experience to identify smaller-than-normal lacrimal glands, this can be learned readily by examining the lacrimal glands of normal patients. Recording lacrimal gland size as normal, small, or atrophic is adequate.

Slit-lamp examination should be done in a consistent, orderly fashion, examining the marginal tear strip, the eyelid margin and lashes, the puncta, and the palpebral and bulbar conjunctiva, concluding with the cornea. Examination of the fornices and the conjunctiva of the everted upper eyelid should be a part of every evaluation.

The height of the marginal tear strip of tear meniscus is noted. Normal height is approximately 0.3 mm. The tear meniscus and preocular tear film are examined also for the presence of mucin debris. In the normal eye, mucin debris usually is absent. The position of the eyelids is noted. Is ectropion or entropion present? The puncta are examined for any enlargement. Frequently, following removal of silicone punctal plugs, the puncta are much larger than normal and may be responsible for increased tear drainage. Are all the puncta present or are they occluded? Are there accessory puncta present? These can result in increased tear drainage. Are the puncta in normal position or are they everted? Misdirected puncta can result in epiphora.

The eyelid margins are examined for thickening, telangiectasis, and irregularity, which suggest chronic blepharitis. Broken and missing eyelashes are found in cases of chronic blepharitis. Trichiasis is usually seen in more severe forms of eyelid inflammation. The presence of scurf suggests seborrheic blepharitis, whereas collarettes suggest staphylococcal blepharitis. The health of the meibomian glands must be assessed. Pouting, plugged, or missing meibomian gland orifices, toothpaste-like secretions, or the presence of oil or foam suggest meibomian gland dysfunction. The presence of segmental inflammation of the posterior eyelid margins suggests meibomianitis.

The bulbar conjunctiva is examined for the presence of papillae, follicles, symblepharon, subepithelial fibrosis, concretions, and injection. The palpebral conjunctiva is examined for the presence of scarring and papillae, and the size and location of the papillae are noted. A papillary reaction involving the inferior palpebral conjunctiva is seen in patients with ocular cicatricial pemphigoid and Sjögren's syndrome. The causes of conjunctivitis involving the upper eyelid are generally limited to SLK, atopic eye disease, vernal, giant papillary conjunctivitis, floppy eyelid syndrome, and trachoma.

The cornea is examined for the presence of adherent mucin and filaments, which are seen in more severe cases of KCS. Patients with filaments usually have a significant decrease in lacrimal gland secretion, increased inflammation, incomplete eyelid closure, or poor "wiper" action of the eyelids. In patients with KCS, filaments form inferiorly where the incomplete blink stops. The presence of corneal irregularity, punctate epithelial erosions, or punctate epithelial keratopathy is noted. Corneal findings are usually noted in patients with more severe KCS or with keratitis medicamentosa due to preservative or medication toxicity. Episcleritis, scleritis, and iridocyclitis can be seen in patients with Sjögren's syndrome and collagen vascular disease. Finally, a baseline intraocular pressure should be obtained in all patients if possible, as patients may be using or may require topical or systemic corticosteroids.

■ Clinical Tests

Measurement of Tear Secretion

Schirmer's and Jones's Tests Unfortunately, the Schirmer's test often is used as the basis (often the only basis) for diagnosis of the dry eye. Originally, this test was introduced to quantify reflex tearing due to conjunctival (Schirmer's I), nasal (Schirmer's II), and retinal stimulation (Schirmer's III) [9]. Jones's basal secretion test used topical anesthesia to eliminate reflex stimulation of tearing [10] but, because topical anesthetics cause irritation and resultant reflex tearing, Jones suggested waiting 2 minutes after topical anesthetic application before performing the test. These tests all use a filter paper strip with a folded end placed between the lower eyelid and globe. The paper should be placed either temporal or nasal to the cornea to avoid corneal irritation and further reflex tearing. Even with topical anesthesia, there is a rapid initial wetting phase lasting 1 to 2 minutes due to absorption of the tear reservoir and local irritation. Over the next 3 to 5 minutes, there is a slower, more linear wetting rate [11]. The most variability occurs in the first 2 minutes. Therefore, readings taken at the end of 2 or 2½ minutes will have a higher rate of wetting than those taken after 5 minutes. Doubling the reading at 2½ minutes may yield erroneously high results. These tests are indirect measures of lacrimal gland secretion, measuring fluid from the tear lake after the fluid has moved across the surface of the eye. They are also subject to the effects of temperature, humidity, and evaporation [12].

Controversy surrounds the issue of which is the best test to use, Schirmer's or Jones's. To determine the maximum amount of tear secretion, use a Schirmer's test without anesthesia, whereas to determine the minimum amount of tear secretion, use Jones's basal tear secretion test. For example, in patients with moderate to severe KCS, where it is important to determine whether a functional lacrimal gland is present, use a Schirmer's test. In suspected mild KCS or contact lens–induced dry eye, where it is important to determine the basal level of tear production, Jones's test is more appropriate.

A standard technique should be used (Table 6). Normal values with and without anesthesia are more than 5 mm of wetting over 5 minutes

Table 6 *Technique for Performing Schirmer's Test*

If topical anesthesia is used, wait 1–2 minutes.
Gently blot fornix.
Place test strip at junction of lateral and middle one-third of lower eyelid.
Dim room lights and allow patient to blink normally.
Measure amount of wetting (in millimeters) after 5 minutes.

and more than 10 mm of wetting, respectively. *These tests should not be used as the only basis of diagnosing KCS.*

Cotton Thread Test A crimped end of a piece of phenol red–impregnated fine cotton thread is placed between the eyelid and globe and the amount of wetting measured over 15 seconds [13]. Normal values are 9 to 18 mm. This test probably measures the volume of the tear lake and not tear flow. Cotton thread test values are not correlated with Schirmer's test values.

Peritron Originally used to estimate gingival fluid flow by electrical conductance, the Peritron has been used also to measure tear volume [14]. This instrument has recently been reintroduced under the name *Tear Tec* (Jerlin Corp., Kansas City, MO). It has poor sensitivity in diagnosing KCS.

Fluorophotometry Using fluorophotometry, it is possible to evaluate tear flow and tear volume by measuring the decay of sodium fluorescein in the tear film after its topical application. By this method, normal tear flow is 0.5 to 2.2 µl/min and normal tear volume 4 to 13 µl [15]. Corneal permeability can also be measured by fluorophotometric techniques. It has been shown that corneal epithelial permeability is 2.8 times greater in patients with dry eye compared to non-dry-eye patients [16].

Measurement of Tear Stability

Fluorescein or Invasive Tear Breakup Time The time elapsed from the blink to appearance of the first random dry spot after application of topical fluorescein to the ocular surface is called the tear breakup time (TBUT) [17]. It is a measurement of the stability of the tear film–ocular surface interface and is almost always abnormal in patients with moderate to severe KCS. A standard technique should be used (Table 7). Normal values are 10 seconds or more. TBUT is decreased during the estrogen phase of the menstrual cycle and by topical anesthetics, preservatives, and ocular ointments [18]. It is increased by application of artificial tears and is unaffected by temperature and humidity.

Table 7 *Technique for Measuring Fluorescein Tear Breakup Time (TBUT)*

Apply several drops of unpreserved solution to a fluorescein strip.
Gently touch the strip to the inferior tear meniscus.
Ask patient to blink and roll eyes around several times.
Wait 1 minute.
Ask patient to close and then keep open his or her eyes.
Measure (in seconds) the time between eye opening and appearance of the first dry spot.
Record the mean of three trials.

Noninvasive TBUT To evaluate TBUT noninvasively, an instrument called a *xeroscope*, which projects rings of light onto the anterior corneal surface, can be used. The time elapsed from blink to distortion of the light rings is measured. A keratometer may also be used. Normal values for noninvasive TBUT are greater than 20 seconds [19].

Measurement of Tear Film Integrity

Of all the clinical tests available, rose bengal staining is the most useful and must be part of every dry-eye workup. It has traditionally been taught that rose bengal is a vital dye that stains dead and dying cells. Recent evidence has shown that rose bengal actually stains areas where the tear film is discontinuous [20]. Rose bengal in a 1% solution is preferable to the impregnated strips.

When placed in the eye (especially in patients with KCS), this dye causes stinging. Therefore, small amounts (5 μl) and a standard technique should be used (Table 8). Areas of staining are scored on a scale of 0 to 3 for the nasal and temporal conjunctiva and cornea, for a total possible score of 9 for each eye [21], although other scoring systems may be used. Scores of 3 or higher are consistent with KCS.

The location of staining can also be a clue to the cause of a dry eye. Interpalpebral bulbar conjunctival and corneal staining is seen in KCS. Inferior corneal staining is seen in trauma, from factious causes, lagoph-

Table 8 *Technique for Rose Bengal Staining*

Apply 5 μl rose bengal to the superior bulbar conjunctiva.
Ask the patient to blink several times and roll the eyes around.
Wait 1 minute.
After 1 minute, use the red-free (green) filter on the slit lamp to examine the conjunctiva and cornea.
Record staining on a scale of 0 to 3 for both the nasal and temporal conjunctiva and cornea.

thalmos, and toxic keratitis. Superior corneal and limbic staining is seen in SLK. Staining of the plica semilunaris and caruncle suggest mucus-fishing syndrome or eye rubbing. The entire cornea stains in severe KCS, in ocular surface diseases such as ocular cicatricial pemphigoid and Stevens-Johnson syndrome and in keratitis medicamentosa. In KCS, the conjunctiva stains earlier in the disease process, whereas the cornea stains as the disease worsens. In ocular surface diseases and keratitis medicamentosa, the cornea stains before the conjunctiva.

Measurement of Epithelial Integrity

Fluorescein stains areas of epithelial cell loss and may actually be a vital dye. Sterile fluorescein-impregnated strips or a 2% solution can be used. A drop of fluorescein is applied to the inferior marginal tear strip, and the patient is asked to blink and roll the eyes to ensure mixing. The amount of conjunctival and corneal staining can be graded similarly to rose bengal scoring or on a scale of 0 to 4+. As with rose bengal dye, conjunctival staining occurs in mild to moderate KCS and corneal staining in more severe KCS.

■ Laboratory Tests

Physical Characteristics of the Tear Film

Tear Film Osmolality The osmolality of the tear film has been shown to be elevated in patients with decreased tear film secretion, increased evaporation, and increased ocular surface exposure (e.g., exophthalmos). As reflex tearing decreases tear film osmolality, nonstimulated tears must be collected. A commercially available osmometer (Clifton Technical Physics, Hartford, NY) is capable of measuring the osmolarity on nanoliter tear samples using freezing-point depression [22]. Values in excess of 312 mosm/kg are consistent with the diagnosis of KCS. Collection (reflex tearing), storage (evaporation), and measurement errors can occur, so meticulous technique is mandatory [23].

Tear Film pH A cyclical variation in tear film pH exists, with an alkaline shift during awake hours and an acidic shift during sleep [24]. The pH in eyes of normal subjects and those with KCS is not significantly different [25].

Ferning Fluids containing electrolytes and protein produce a fernlike pattern when placed on a glass slide and allowed to dry. Cervical secretions, tears, and other body fluids can form fern patterns [26]. The ferning test consists of placing a drop of tear fluid on a glass slide and allowing it to dry. The presence or absence of ferning is noted. Various schemes can be used to grade the ferning pattern, but ferning does not correlate with other dry-eye tests, and its significance is not known.

Tear Film Evaporation   In patients with KCS, tear film evaporation rates are increased to values twice those of normal subjects [27]. Measurement requires special goggles and instrumentation.

Chemical Composition of the Tear Film

Electrolyte Composition   Sodium and potassium concentrations can be measured in tears using atomic absorption spectrometry. The electrolyte composition of tears in patients with KCS may be abnormal [28].

Protein Composition   Electrophoresis can be used to separate the various proteins in tears. The electrophoretic pattern of tears from normal subjects and patients with KCS show qualitative differences [29].

Lysozyme   Tear film lysozyme levels are the same for men and women and account for 20 to 40% of the total tear protein. Tear film lysozyme levels decrease with age and are reduced in patients using practolol and in those with KCS. Lysozyme levels can be measured by a variety of biochemical techniques, including electroimmunodiffusion, enzyme-linked immunosorbent assay, radial immunodiffusion, agar diffusion, and turbidimetric assays. A commercially available bacteriolytic assay (Quantiplate, Kalstead, Chaska, MN), which estimates lysozyme concentrations indirectly, is available [30]. Tear lysozyme levels of less than 1 mg/ml are consistent with the diagnosis of KCS.

Lactoferrin   One-fourth of the protein in reflex tears is lactoferrin, and it is twice as plentiful in the tears of normal subjects compared to patients with KCS. Lactoferrin chelates iron and interacts with lysozyme and IgA to provide an antimicrobial defense in the tear film. A commercially available radial immunodiffusion assay is available (Lactoplate, Eagle Vision, Memphis, TN) [31]. Tear fluid is collected by placing a circular filter paper 4 mm in diameter in the inferior cul-de-sac. Topical anesthesia is not used. The paper discs are removed, blotted, and placed on the agar gel, which is impregnated with antibody to tear lactoferrin. After 72 hours, a visible precipitate appears. Lactoferrin concentration is proportional to the square of the diameter of the precipitant ring. Normal levels exceed 1 mg/ml.

Histological Evaluation

Ocular Surface   The bulbar conjunctival surface consists of epithelial and goblet cells. Conjunctival scrapings, washings, cutting biopsy, and impression cytology can be used to obtain cells for evaluation. In KCS, the bulbar conjunctival surface undergoes squamous metaplasia, with resultant keratinization of the epithelial cells and loss of goblet cells. Scrapings and washings yield individual cells and cell clumps. Cutting biopsy allows evaluation of the conjunctiva in cross section. Conjunctival impression cytology (CIC) removes one to three layers of the surface conjunctival epithelium and goblet cells. Cutting biopsy is required to determine basement membrane deposition of IgG, IgM, and complement in patients with ocular cicatricial pemphigoid.

Conjunctival Impression Cytology For CIC, specimens are obtained from the nasal and temporal interpalpebral and superior bulbar conjunctiva and the inferior palpebral conjunctiva. Circular discs or strips of cellulose acetate filter material are pressed onto the conjunctival surface for 2 seconds. An ophthalmodynanometer is used to apply a standardized pressure of 40 gm to the bulbar conjunctival surface and 70 gm to the inferior palpebral surface. Specimens are then carefully removed, fixed, and stained using periodic acid–Schiff stain to stain goblet cell mucin and hematoxylin as a counterstain. Next the specimens are dried and coverslipped. Each specimen is graded (0 through 3) according to the number of goblet cells present and the degree of epithelial cell abnormality. Grade 0 specimens have normal numbers of goblet cells and normal-appearing epithelial cells, whereas grade 3 specimens have no goblet cells and keratinized epithelial cells. Any specimen with a grade higher than 1 is considered abnormal. In KCS, the bulbar conjunctival surface is abnormal (grade > 1), whereas the inferior palpebral conjunctival surface is normal (grade ≤ 1) [32, 33]. Although CIC is useful in diagnosing KCS, there are regional conjunctival surface and normal variations that can make interpretation difficult. Because this technique removes only one to three layers of cells, it is not a substitute for a flat-mounted preparation.

Lacrimal Gland Biopsy Biopsy of the lacrimal gland is not difficult to perform and can yield information that may be helpful in the diagnosis of Sjögren's syndrome. However, minor salivary gland involvement often is found in cases of lacrimal gland involvement, and biopsy of the minor salivary glands generally is sufficient. On histological examination, the presence of more than 1 aggregate of 50 lymphocytes/4 mm^2 (focus score > 1) is consistent with a diagnosis of Sjögren's syndrome. Biopsy is done under topical anesthesia followed by a superotemporal subconjunctival injection of 2% lidocaine with epinephrine. The palpebral lobe of the lacrimal gland is prolapsed and an incision made through the conjunctiva and capsule. A small piece of tissue is removed and placed in fixative. There is usually minimal bleeding, and no suturing is required.

Minor Salivary Gland (Labial or Lip) Biopsy Biopsy of the minor salivary glands of the lower lip is very helpful in the diagnosis of Sjögren's syndrome, and it is probably safer and more convenient than lacrimal gland biopsy. A focus score exceeding 1 is consistent with a diagnosis of Sjögren's syndrome. The procedure is not difficult and is well tolerated. Cotton-tipped applicators, saturated with topical ophthalmic anesthetic, are applied to one side of the median raphe of the lower lip. An injection of 2% lidocaine with epinephrine is given submucosally. A large chalazion clamp is applied to the lip to control bleeding. An incision is made through the mucosa until the minor salivary glands prolapse into the wound. Five gland lobules are removed and placed in fixative. The wound is closed with a running submucosal suture of 4-0 or 6-0 chromic catgut.

■ Response to Treatment Trials

Often a treatment trial will aid in diagnosis of the dry eye. Treatment with artificial lubricants will result in one of three responses—improvement, worsening, or no change. Patients with keratitis medicamentosa due to preservatives improve with discontinuation of preservatives and nonpreserved artificial lubricants. Patients with moderate to severe KCS usually improve with very frequent use of topical nonpreserved lubricants, whereas patients with milder disease may worsen with frequent artificial lubricants due to washing out of their own tears. If inflammation is present, patients may require topical steroids (nonpreserved, if possible) for improvement. Oral tetracycline usually results in significant improvement in patients with rosacea blepharitis. Patients with blepharospasm respond dramatically to botulinum toxin (Botox, Allergan Pharmaceuticals, Irvine, CA).

■ Findings in Specific Dry-Eye Syndromes

A suggested office workup of the dry eye is shown in Table 9. A brief discussion of the historical and clinical findings of several dry-eye diseases follows. Knowledge of these findings may aid the ophthalmologist in differentiating KCS from other dry-eye conditions.

Keratoconjunctivitis Sicca

History Patients with KCS present with symptoms of foreign-body sensation, burning, dryness, and photophobia. Curiously, patients with Sjögren's syndrome have increased photophobia in fluorescent-lighted envi-

Table 9 *Office Workup of the Dry Eye*

History
Symptoms history: burning, foreign-body sensation, itching, mattering, photophobia, irritant and emotional tearing
Topical lubricant history
Topical and systemic medications
Review of systems: xerostomia, decreased vaginal secretions, joint pain, fatigue
Systemic diseases: lupus erythematosus, rheumatoid arthritis, Sjögren's syndrome and other collagen vascular diseases, thyroid disease

Clinical examination
External
    Visual assessment of patient
    Salivary and thyroid glands, hands and facial skin
    Tear meniscus
    Schirmer's test (without anesthesia)
    Eyelids: blink rate, closure, lagophthalmos
    Jones's basal secretion test (with anesthesia)

Slit lamp
    Eyelids: blepharitis, ectropion, entropion, punctal size and position, trichiasis
    Conjunctiva and cornea: increased mucin, filaments, punctate staining, ulceration
    Tear breakup time
    Fluorescein staining
    Rose bengal staining

ronments. Symptoms are least on awakening and worsen as the day progresses. Systemic diseases such as RA, SLE, or other collagen vascular diseases may suggest Sjögren's syndrome. Xerostomia, decreased vaginal secretions, fatigue, and KCS suggest Sjögren's syndrome. Hypothyroidism may be present. Most patients will have used artificial lubricants with some relief. Those with severe disease will have worsening of symptoms with preserved lubricants. Patients may be using systemic medications that decrease tear secretion.

Clinical Examination On slit-lamp examination, the marginal tear strip will be decreased. In more severe disease, mucin debris in the tear film and corneal filaments may be present. The results of Schirmer's test (with anesthesia) and Jones's basal tear secretion test will be decreased from normal. TBUT will be 10 seconds or less. Rose bengal staining scores will be 3 or more out of 9, with interpalpebral staining of the conjunctiva. Corneal staining will be seen in more severe disease, and there is increased discomfort with corneal involvement.

Laboratory and Histological Evaluation Tear lactoferrin and lysozyme levels are decreased (<1 mg/ml) and tear film osmolality increased (>312 mosm/L) in KCS. By CIC, there is an abnormal bulbar conjunctiva (grade > 1) and a normal inferior palpebral conjunctiva. Lacrimal and minor salivary gland biopsies are positive, with a focus score higher than 1 in patients with Sjögren's syndrome.

Blepharitis

History Patients with blepharitis present with symptoms of burning and mattering on awakening. Symptoms are worse on awakening, better within an hour or so, and worse again later in the day. Patients may have rosacea or seborrheic dermatitis. There is minimal response to artificial lubricants, but eyelid hygiene done on a chronic basis improves symptoms. Oral tetracycline also may improve symptoms and signs, especially in rosacea blepharitis.

Clinical Examination In posterior marginal blepharitis, there is meibomian gland dysfunction, with oil on the eyelid margins, plugged meibomian duct orifices, and inspissated glands. In anterior margin blepharitis, there may be collarettes (staphylococcal) or scurf (seborrheic). Often, poor or incomplete blinking is present. There may be inflammation of the meibomian glands (meibomianitis) and increased tear film debris, as well as inferior punctate corneal staining with fluorescein. TBUT usually is abnormal. If tear secretion is decreased and interpalpebral rose bengal staining is present, there may be coexistent KCS.

Laboratory and Histological Evaluation Tear film osmolality is increased in blepharitis. CIC usually shows abnormal bulbar and palpebral conjunctival surfaces.

Toxic or Irritant Keratoconjunctivitis

History Patients with toxic or irritant keratoconjunctivitis present with symptoms of burning, foreign-body sensation, and photophobia, which are present all the time and worsen with continued use of the offending agent or in the offending environment. There may be a history of KCS. Often, a patient begins using a preserved lubricant four to six times daily. Then, as symptoms increase, more frequent application becomes necessary. A vicious cycle develops as the patient increases the frequency of drop usage to relieve symptoms that are aggravated by the preservative in the lubricant.

Clinical Examination Findings in this form of keratoconjunctivitis are mostly corneal unless KCS also is present. There is punctate staining of the entire corneal surface, and filaments may be present.

Laboratory and Histological Evaluation Findings on laboratory and histological workup are usually consistent with the underlying disease, if any. CIC evaluation shows abnormal bulbar and palpebral conjunctival surfaces and the presence of polymorphonuclear leukocytes.

Allergic Keratoconjunctivitis

History Symptoms of allergic keratoconjunctivitis are primarily itching and mattering. Symptoms may follow a pattern, as in seasonal hayfever keratoconjunctivitis or environmental exposure. A history of hay fever or atopic dermatitis often is present.

Clinical Examination A papillary conjunctivitis is present. In atopic eye disease, giant papillary conjunctivitis, and vernal keratoconjunctivitis, papillae of various sizes are present on the upper palpebral conjunctiva. There may be mucin debris in the tear film. However, there is usually no rose bengal or fluorescein staining present unless the papillae are large enough to cause mechanical injury to the cornea.

Laboratory and Histological Evaluation In allergic keratoconjunctivitis, eosinophils may be seen on conjunctival scrapings.

Ocular Surface Diseases

History Patients with ocular surface disease—ocular cicatricial pemphigoid, lichen planus, and Stevens-Johnson syndrome—usually present with a chronic, recurrent conjunctivitis. Symptoms of foreign-body sensation and burning fluctuate with varying intensity during the day and over time, often with reddened eyes and mucous drainage. There may be associated oral and esophageal lesions in ocular cicatricial pemphigoid and skin and oral lesions in Stevens-Johnson syndrome. Also in patients with pemphigoid, there may be a history of antiglaucomatous medication usage.

Clinical Examination Conjunctival inflammation, a papillary conjunctivitis, and conjunctival subepithelial fibrosis are signs of active disease. As the disease progresses, symblepharon form, and trichiasis appears in more severe, chronic disease. The cornea stains with fluorescein earlier in the disease than does the conjunctiva. If the lacrimal gland excretory ducts are obliterated by the cicatrizing process, findings of KCS may be present.

Laboratory and Histological Evaluation Conjunctival biopsy shows basement membrane immunoglobulin deposition of complement, IgG, and IgM in ocular cicatricial pemphigoid. CIC evaluation shows abnormal bulbar and palpebral conjunctival surfaces.

References

1. Lucca JA, Farris RL. Keratoconjunctivitis sicca in male patients with human immunodeficiency virus type I. Ophthalmology 1990;97:1008–1010
2. Calissendorff B, el-A-zazi M, Lonnquist B. Dry eye syndrome in long-term follow-up of bone marrow transplanted patients. Bone Marrow Transplant 1989;4:675–678
3. Vold SD, Carroll RP, Nelson JD. Dermatochalasis and dry eye: a surgically treatable syndrome. Am J Ophthalmol 1993;115:216–220
4. Gilbard JP, Rossi SR, Heyda KG. Tear film and ocular surface changes after closure of the meibomian gland orifices in the rabbit. Ophthalmology 1989;96:1180–1186
5. Lemp MA, Mahmood MA, Weiler HH. Association of rosacea and keratoconjunctivitis sicca. Arch Ophthalmol 1988;105:670–673
6. Pfister RR, Burstein N. The effects of ophthalmic drugs, vehicles and preservatives on corneal epithelium: a scanning electron microscopy study. Invest Ophthalmol Vis Sci 1976;15:246–259
7. Nelson J, Silverman V, Lima P, Anderson-Beckman G. Corneal epithelial wound healing: a tissue culture assay on the effects of antibiotics. Curr Eye Res 1990;9:277–285
8. Wilson FM. Adverse external effects of topical ophthalmic medications. Surv Ophthalmol 1979;24:57–88
9. Schirmer O. Studien zur physiologie und pathologie der tranenabsonderung und tranenabfuhr. Graefes Arch Clin Exp Ophthalmol 1903;56:197–291
10. Jones LT. The lacrimal secretory system and its treatment. Am J Ophthalmol 1966;62:47–60
11. Clinch TE, Benedetto DA, Felberg NT, Laibson PR. Schirmer's test: a closer look. Arch Ophthalmol 1983;101:1383–1386
12. Holly FJ, Esquivel ED. Lacrimation kinetics in humans as determined by a novel technique. In: Holly FJ, ed. The preocular tear film. Lubbock, TX: Dry Eye Institute, 1986:76–88
13. Hamano H, Hori M, Hamono T, et al. A new method for measuring tears. CLAO J 1983;9:281–289
14. Farris RL, Gilbard JP, Stuchell RN, Mandell ID. Diagnostic tests in keratoconjunctivitis sicca. CLAO J 1983;9:23–28
15. Göbbels M, Goebels G, Britbach R, Spitznas M. Tear secretion in dry eyes as assessed by objective fluorophotometry. Ger J Ophthalmol 1992;1:350–353
16. Göbbels M, Spitznas M. Influence of artificial tears on corneal epithelium in dry-eye syndrome. Graefes Arch Clin Exp Ophthalmol 1989;227:139–141
17. Norn MS. Desiccation of the precorneal tear film. I. Corneal wetting time. Acta Ophthalmol (Copenh) 1969;47:865–880
18. Lemp MA, Hamill JR. Factors affecting tear breakup in normal eyes. Arch Ophthalmol 1973;89:103–105
19. Mengher LS, Bron AJ, Tonge SR, Gilbert DJ. A non-invasive instrument for clinical assessment of the pre-corneal tear film stability. Curr Eye Res 1985;4:9–12
20. Feenstra RPC, Tseng SCG. What is actually stained by rose bengal? Arch Ophthalmol 1992;110:984–993

21. van Bijsterveld OP. Diagnostic tests in the sicca syndrome. Arch Ophthalmol 1969; 82:10–14
22. Farris RL, Stuchell RN, Mandel ID. Basal and reflex human tear analysis I. Physical measurements: osmolarity, basal volumes, and reflex flow rate. Ophthalmology 1981;88:852–857
23. Nelson JD, Wright JC. Tear film osmolality determination: an evaluation of potential errors in measurement. Curr Eye Res 1986;5:677–681
24. Carney LG, Hill RM. Human tear pH: diurnal variations. Arch Ophthalmol 1976; 94:821–824
25. Browning DJ, Foulks GN. Tear pH in health, disease and contact lens wear. In: Holly FJ, ed. The preocular tear film. Lubbock, TX: Dry Eye Institute, 1986: 954–965
26. Tabbara KF, Okumoto M. A qualitative test for mucus deficiency. Ophthalmology 1982;89:712–714
27. Rolando M, Refojo MF, Kenyon KR. Increased tear evaporation in eyes with keratoconjunctivitis sicca. Arch Ophthalmol 1983;101:557–558
28. Gilbard JP, Rossi SR. An electrolyte-based solution that increases corneal glycogen and conjunctival goblet-cell density in a rabbit model for keratoconjunctivitis sicca. Ophthalmology 1992;99:600–604
29. Boukes RJ, Boonstra A, Breebaart AC, et al. Analysis of human tear protein profiles using high performance liquid chromatography (HPLC). Doc Ophthalmol 1987;67: 105–113
30. van Bijsterveld OP. Standardization of the lysozyme test for a commercially available medium. Arch Ophthalmol 1974;91:432–434
31. van Bijsterveld OP. A simple test for lacrimal gland function: a tear lactoferrin assay by radial immunodiffusion. Graefes Arch Clin Exp Ophthalmol 1983;220:171–174
32. Nelson JD. Impression cytology. Cornea 1988;7:71–81
33. Nelson JD. Diagnostic impression cytology in contact lens wear. In: Diabezies O, ed. Contact lenses: CLAO guide to basic science and clinical practice. Boston: Little, Brown, 1989:3C1–3C7

Evaluation of the Ocular Surface in Dry-Eye Conditions

Scheffer C. G. Tseng, M.D., Ph.D.

■ Relationship Between Ocular Surface Epithelia and Preocular Tear Film

Stable Preocular Tear Film Protects Ocular Surface Epithelia

The normal ocular surface is covered by a thin layer of tear film. A stable tear film ensures comfort while serving as an effective refractive optical surface for vision while the eye is open. As the first line of defense against microbial infections, a stable tear film also maintains healthy ocular surface epithelia (corneal, limbal, and conjunctival) [1, 2].

Tear film stability has developed through evolution to include several protective mechanisms [3]. These protective mechanisms, inherent in external adnexa and outlined in Table 1, can be grossly subdivided into two major types: compositional and hydrodynamic. It is generally believed that the precorneal tear film is composed of a superficial thin lipid layer (primarily derived from meibum excreted by meibomian glands), a middle bulky aqueous layer (consisting of proteins, electrolytes, and water secreted mainly by lacrimal glands), and an innermost mucus layer (derived from mucins secreted by conjunctival goblet cells). Aside from these layered tear components, the tear film is controlled by hydrodynamic factors. Tears are mechanically spread over the ocular surface through a neuronally controlled eyelid-blinking mechanism, driven by the intact corneal sensitivity. Also through blinking, the old used tears are cleared from the ocular surface via a patent nasolacrimal drainage duct into the nose.

Ocular Surface Epithelia Play an Active Role in Maintaining Tear Film Stability

From a physical point of view, formation of a thin preocular tear film requires the lowering of tensions at two interfaces [1, 2]. At the air-fluid interface, it is achieved by the superficial lipid layer, whereas at the fluid-cell interface, it is ensured by the mucus layer [1, 2]. Mucus is a gel found in most wet epithelial surfaces and acts as a medium for protection, lubrication, and transport. Mucins, the primary component of mucus gels, are large proteins and highly glycosylated glycoproteins with polydispersity and heterogeneity [4, 5].

All biochemical characterization of ocular mucins has been performed using mucoid clots collected from inferior forniceal conjunctiva [6–10]. Owing to insufficient material, no mucin characterization has been performed directly on the preocular mucus layer. From the ocular surface bathing fluid, my colleagues and I purified and characterized rabbit ocular mucin and noted that there were at least three mucin fractions [11]. Since the concept of layered tear components was introduced by Wolff in 1954 [12], it has been believed that the precorneal mucus layer is derived from conjunctival goblet cells because the corneal epithelium does not contain goblet cells. Using a polyclonal antibody to mucins purified from mucoid clots, Moore and Tiffany [7] showed that the source of mucoid clots is conjunctival goblet cells and not lacrimal glands, but it remains unclear whether the mucoid clots are indeed a turnover product directly derived from the precorneal tear film. Although polyanionic glycoconjugates, sometimes called *glycocalyx*, are present on the corneal [13–17] and conjunctival [13–21] surface, their identity remains obscure.

Previously, we developed several monoclonal antibodies to conjunctival goblet cell–secreted mucin (GCM) ([22]; also MM Mui and SCG Tseng, unpublished report). To our surprise, one of them—AM3—of which the antigenic epitope has been characterized to be in the nonglycosylated peptide domain, vividly stains conjunctival goblet cells but does not stain the precorneal mucus layer (Fig 1). As this paradoxical negative result could not be attributed to the poor preservation of precorneal tear film, we searched for and discovered mucosal epithelium–associated mucinlike glycoproteins (MEM) by two newly developed monoclonal antibodies, AMEM1 and AMEM2 [23]. An immunofluorescence tissue survey reveals that its antigenic epitope is distributed in nearly all wet mucosa of digestive, respiratory, and urogenital tracts. In the conjunctival epithelium, MEM was expressed by goblet and nongoblet epithelial cells. Interestingly, in the corneal epithelium, MEM was expressed as punctate, filamentous structures on the membrane of the two superficial epithelial layers (see Fig 1) [24]. A double-labeling immunofluorescence study shows that the antigenic epitope of MEM does not codistribute with that of GCM. MEM also differs from GCM in aqueous solubility, N-acetylcysteine extractability, and acetylcholine dischargeability [24].

Taken together, these data strongly suggest that there are at least two types of ocular mucins defined by immunoreactivity and that the precorneal tear film predominantly consists of a unique type of MEM that can exist in membranous and extracellular (secreted) forms. These findings

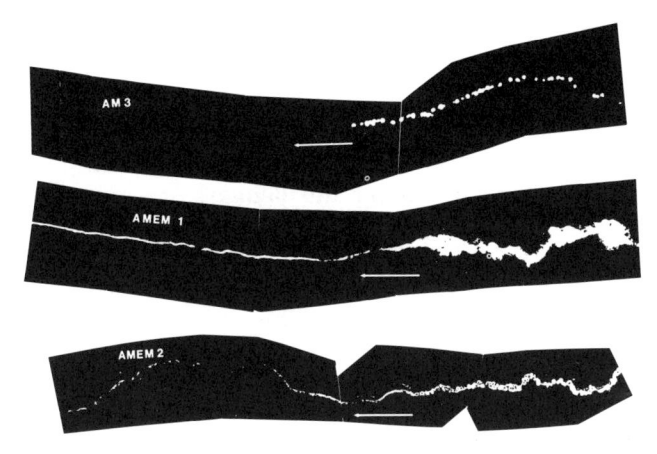

Figure 1 Immunofluorescence staining of rabbit ocular surface epithelia with three monoclonal antibodies. AM3, which recognizes conjunctival goblet cell–secreted mucin, stains all conjunctival goblet cells but not the precorneal mucus layer. In contrast, AMEM1 and AMEM2, which recognize mucosal epithelium–associated mucinlike glycoproteins, stain goblet cells as well as the superficial layers of nongoblet epithelial cells, of which the latter are also noted in the precorneal mucus layer. The same result is noted on human ocular surface. Bars indicate the limbal regions, with arrows pointing to the corneal side.

also lead to a new concept that nongoblet epithelial cells of cornea and conjunctiva play an active role in maintaining the tear film stability. It is likely that MEM expressed by nongoblet epithelial cells can interact with GCM secreted by conjunctival goblet cells and, through this mucin interaction, the interfacial tension between tear fluid and epithelial cell membrane is lowered and tear film is thus stabilized. This new concept suggests that in addition to compositional and hydrodynamic factors, tear film stability is controlled by the ocular surface epithelia via their normal terminal differentiation (see Table 1).

Table 1 Protective Mechanisms Ensuring Tear Film Stability

Preocular tear film
1. Compositional factors
   a. Lipid tear: produced primarily by meibomian glands
   b. Aqueous tear: produced primarily by lacrimal glands
   c. Mucus tear: believed to be produced by conjunctival goblet cells
2. Hydrodynamic factors
   a. Corneal sensitivity*
   b. Mechanical spread via eyelid blinking
   c. Clearance via eyelid blinking (pump) and a smooth passage

Ocular surface epithelia

*Corneal sensitivity controls 1.b, 2.b, and 2.c.

Clinical Evaluation of the Ocular Surface in Dry Eyes

Tear film stability can be threatened by many dry-eye disorders that disturb the compositional and hydrodynamic aspects of the protective mechanisms. An unstable tear film is the hallmark of various dry-eye states. Because the term *unstable tear film* conveys the pathogenesis better than the common term *dry eyes*, these terms are used interchangeably in this chapter.

As we have just established, the ocular surface epithelia are protected by stable preocular tear film; in turn, the ocular surface epithelia play an active role in maintaining tear film stability. Hence, alteration of either of these will likely affect the other.

Clinically, a number of functional tests of tears have been employed to evaluate the status of preocular tear film and tear film stability. Among these are tear breakup time (invasive and noninvasive), Schirmer's tests (anesthetized, unanesthetized, or stimulated), the tear clearance test, measurements of tear protein components (e.g., lysozyme, lactoferrin), and measurements of various physiochemical properties of tears (e.g., evaporation, osmolarity). Because many of these tear tests will be described in other chapters in this issue, they will not be elaborated here. Clinically, two tests that can be used to evaluate ocular surface epithelia are dye staining and impression cytology. Impression cytology is described by other authors in this issue, so my focus will be on dye staining and the cytological findings relevant to dye staining.

Vital Dye Staining

The concept of vital dye staining, first introduced by Ehrlich in 1886, describes the staining by a dye of cells, bacteria, protozoa, or tissues in their living state. A dye exhibiting this property is called a *vital dye*, four of which have been used or reported to be useful for the diagnosis of various ocular surface disorders. These are fluorescein, rose bengal, lissamine green B, and sulforhodamine B. Their respective chemical structures are shown in Figure 2.

The use of rose bengal, the 4,5,6,7-tetrachloro-2′,4′,5′,7′-tetraiodo derivative of fluorescein, has been greatly promoted ever since Sjögren [25] in 1933 described a unique staining pattern by rose bengal for patients with keratoconjunctivitis sicca syndrome. Without direct evidence, Sjögren [25], and later Passmore and King [26], speculated that rose bengal stained desquamated epithelial cells. It was not until between 1962 and 1972 that Norn [27, 28] established that rose bengal does not stain normal healthy epithelial cells but stains dead or degenerated cells and mucous strands. Based on this concept, 1% rose bengal has been clinically adopted to establish the diagnosis of keratoconjunctivitis sicca in Sjögren's syndrome in several earlier and recent studies (e.g., [29]). This concept has been ex-

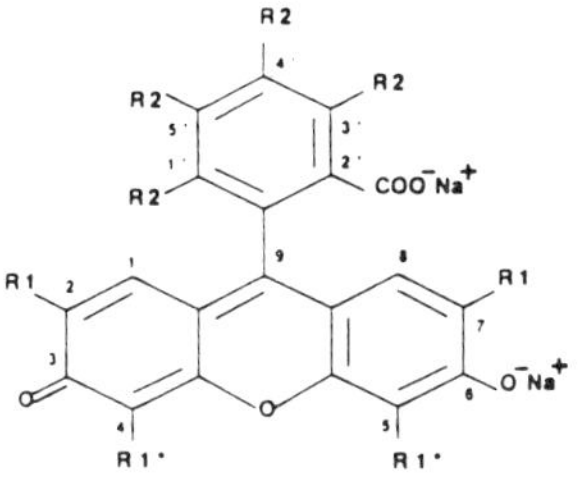

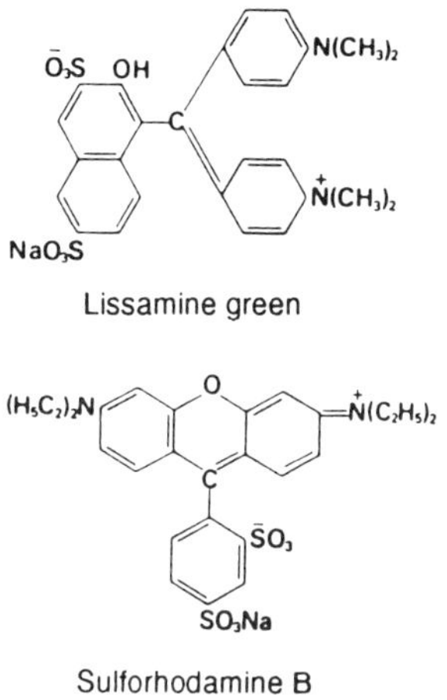

Figure 2 *Chemical structures of fluorescein, rose bengal, sulforhodamine B, and lissamine green B. Fluorescein and rose bengal belong to the hydroxyxanthene dye family and sulforhodamine B to the aminoxanthene dye family. Note that rose bengal has a high content of halides, but sulforhodamine B and lissamine green B have amino and sulfate groups. Fluorescein is devoid of any of these functional groups.*

tended also to interpret other lesions such as epithelial dendrites of herpes simplex and zoster [30], dysplasia or squamous metaplasia of conjunctival squamous neoplasms [31], and various forms of superficial punctate keratitis [32].

While exploring the mechanism of photothrombosis, a novel technique for occluding blood vessels using intravenous injection of rose bengal and argon green laser irradiation [33], my colleagues and I noted that rose bengal was instantly taken up by several types of healthy cultured cells [34]. Prompted by this surprising finding, we reexamined the accuracy of this current concept and reported that indeed rose bengal stained healthy cultured [35] and ex vivo [36] corneal epithelium. To explain the mechanism by which the ocular surface epithelium normally is not stained by rose bengal, a well-known fact but paradoxical with respect to our experimental finding, we further demonstrated that such tear components as albumin and mucin effectively block rose bengal uptake [35]. We thus propose that rose bengal's ability to stain is dictated by the status of tear film protection and not by the status of cell vitality.

We then analyzed how different tear components may protect the surface epithelia from rose bengal staining. Two basic mechanisms were identified: strong dye binding, preventing dye uptake by cells, and action as a diffusion barrier in the absence of strong binding, delaying dye uptake [35, 36]. Although experimentally, albumin binds rose bengal strongly and thus prevents cell staining, albumin is not a major tear protein [37]. Measurements of the dissociation constants (Kds) of all major tear proteins binding with rose bengal revealed that if tears consisted only of proteins, their maximal total binding capacity would be negligible and could not account for the blocking effect observed under normal circumstances [38]. In contrast, porcine stomach mucin did not bind rose bengal as does albumin but rather exhibited effective blocking as a diffusion barrier. These data further confirm that mucins play a major role in tear film protection, and rose bengal is a dye ideal for detecting ocular surface epithelia that are not well-protected by the healthy tear film.

Mishima [39] earlier showed that tear fluid retention on the corneal surface is lost when the mucus layer is scraped together with the superficial cell layers (which we know contain MEMs). Holly and Lemp [40] showed that the wettability of the corneal epithelium measured by surface tension is promoted by coating with a layer of porcine submaxillary mucin.

Clinically, the degree of unstable tear film measured by tear film breakup time correlates well with increasing rose bengal staining in a number of dry-eye disorders that are characterized by surface squamous metaplasia together with loss of conjunctival goblet cells [41–43]. Now that we know MEM is expressed by nongoblet surface epithelial cells (see Fig 1), MEM's protective role in precluding rose bengal staining is further supported by a recent corneal explant study (Fig 3). Taken together, these data are sufficient to support the contention that rose bengal is unique for detecting the protective status of preocular tear film.

When the staining property of rose bengal was compared to that of fluorescein, we noted that the addition of more halides in this hydroxyxanthene dye family (see Fig 2) decreases the dye's penetration into corneal stroma and increases the dye's intrinsic cell toxicity and photosensitizing toxicity (Table 2) [35]. These unique properties of rose bengal explain why in topical solution it causes smarting on patients' eyes and has an antiviral effect [44]. Recently, sulforhodamine B [45], an aminoxanthene dye, and previously, lissamine green B [46–48] were reported to be superior to fluorescein and rose bengal, respectively, in the clinical diagnoses of various *conjunctival* epithelial lesions that show disturbances in tear film protection. Unlike the halides in rose bengal, the functional groups in these two dyes are sulfate and amine (see Fig 2), which are commonly found in mucin oligosaccharide chains. Recently, we noted that lissamine green B and sulforhodamine B did not stain healthy conjunctival epithelium even when the surface mucus tear layer was insufficient [49]. The staining characteristics of sulforhodamine B and lissamine green B have been compared further to those of fluorescein and rose bengal [50]. Table 2 summarizes the major differences among these four dyes.

It is important to point out in this table that rose bengal differs from the other three dyes in its rapid staining of healthy cells. This unique property renders rose bengal unqualified or illegible as a vital dye. The

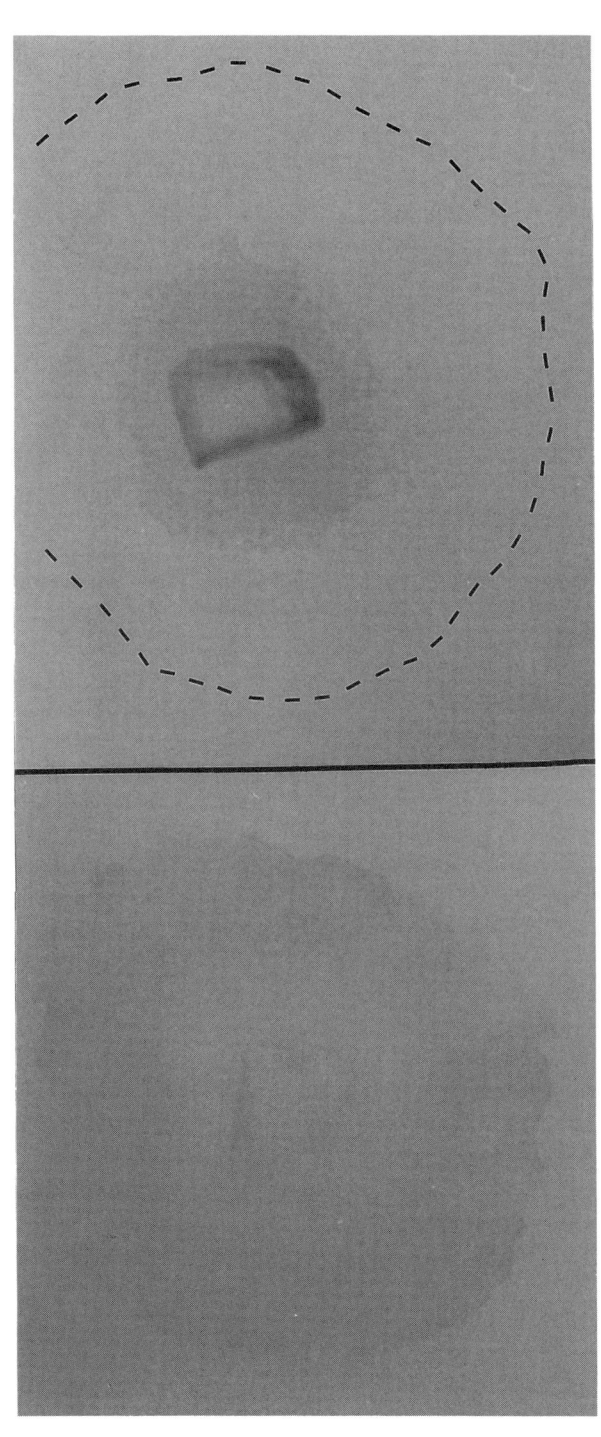

Figure 3 On this rabbit corneal explant epithelial outgrowth, the central periexplant area is positive for MEM expression, as evidenced by positive brown staining with AMEM1, and corresponds with negative rose bengal staining. The peripheral area shows the opposite result.

Table 2 *Summary of Differences Between Four Different Dye Stainings*

	Fluorescein	Rose Bengal	Lissamine Green B	Sulforhodamine B
Experimental				
Stains healthy cells[a]	No	Yes	No	No
Stains dead or degenerative cells	No	Yes	Yes	No[b]
Staining blocked by mucin	No	Yes	No	NA
Intrinsic toxicity	No	Yes	Yes	No
Phototoxicity	No	Yes	ND	No
Relative speed for stromal diffusion	Fastest	Slowest	Fast	Slow
Clinical extrapolation				
Staining promoted by	Disruptions of cell-cell junctions	Insufficient protection by preocular tear film[c]	Cell death or degeneration and disruption of cell-cell junctions	Disruption of cell-cell junctions

NA = not applicable because staining is not detected when cells are dead or degenerative; ND = not done.
[a]Staining is defined by stainability detected by clinical means (i.e., by the naked eye or under a biomicroscope).
[b]Probable yes if appropriate excitation and emission filters are used [45].
[c]Insufficient protection can come from either decreased mucin components or abnormal surface epithelial cells.

added fact that its staining is effectively blocked by the healthy tear mucus layer makes rose bengal the most ideal dye for evaluating the protective status of preocular tear film, a notion first recognized by Sjögren [25]. In contrast, lissamine green B is ideal as a vital dye for detecting dead or degenerative cells. Fluorescein remains the prototypical dye for detecting ocular surface pathological processes mainly manifested as disruption of cell-cell junctions. Sulforhodamine B has properties similar to fluorescein but, for the reasons described by Eliason and Maurice [45], is superior to fluorescein in detecting conjunctival epithelial lesions.

How to Perform Dye Staining

Clinicians must know how to perform dye staining and several key concepts in interpreting the results if they intend to use the stainings effectively for evaluating the ocular surface in various dry-eye conditions. To obtain an interpretable result, it is important to apply an adequate amount of dye because dye staining is concentration-dependent [36]. Commercially, fluorescein and rose bengal are available as drops and strips; only the drops provide a constant concentration. Therefore, variable results are likely to occur when strips are used. Because mechanical (rubbing or touching) or chemical (via anesthetics or preservatives) irritation can induce cellular damage, thus allowing dye to stain those areas, it is imperative to perform the staining prior to some other eye examinations. In this situation, the use of strip wet with preservative-free saline will be better. If anesthetics are to be used with rose bengal stain to avoid the smarting effect, they should be applied immediately before the dye staining. Because rose bengal–stained cells lead to cell death due to the dye's intrinsic toxicity and photosensitizing toxic effects [35], it is advised that the dye be irrigated with preservative-free saline immediately after its application. To ensure that dye is mixed well and has equal access to all ocular surfaces, it is advised that the dye be applied as a drop directly onto the superior bulbar conjunctiva without touching the surface and that the patient be asked to blink several times afterward. Interpretation should be done immediately after dye application because staining is concentration-dependent. As is commonly noted, observation of fluorescein staining is enhanced by blue light, whereas red-free (green) light enhances rose bengal staining. Lissamine green B, though widely used in Europe, is not commercially available in the United States. The usefulness of sulforhodamine B is limited because like lissamine green B, it is not available for clinical use in the United States.

How to Interpret Dye Staining

Differential Use of Dyes As mentioned earlier and summarized in Table 2, different dyes can yield stainings that are not directly comparable. Therefore, it is potentially erroneous to assume that fluorescein staining is the same as rose bengal staining. In dry-eye conditions, ocular surface cells can exhibit squamous metaplasia, a finding confirmed by impression cytology [51–53]. Due to dryness, some squamous metaplastic cells exhibit increased cell desquamation with disruption at the cell-cell junctions; alternatively, they show cellular degeneration or death. The use of topical medication or tear substitutes with preservatives also can cause potentially toxic effects leading to cell desquamation and cell degeneration. Therefore, cellular changes, ranging from loss of cell-cell junctions to poor tear film protection to cell degeneration and death, can all take place in dry-eye conditions, and these will not necessarily occur at the same cell areas. Therefore, fluorescein staining does not necessarily correspond to rose bengal staining and rose bengal staining does not necessarily match with lissamine green staining. Thus we predict that differential use of two or more dyes might yield information for better differential diagnosis. Table 2 can be used as a guide for this purpose. Even for the same dry-eye condition, such combined use of several dye stainings might disclose different underlying pathological insults (e.g., squamous metaplasia versus cell-cell junction disruption).

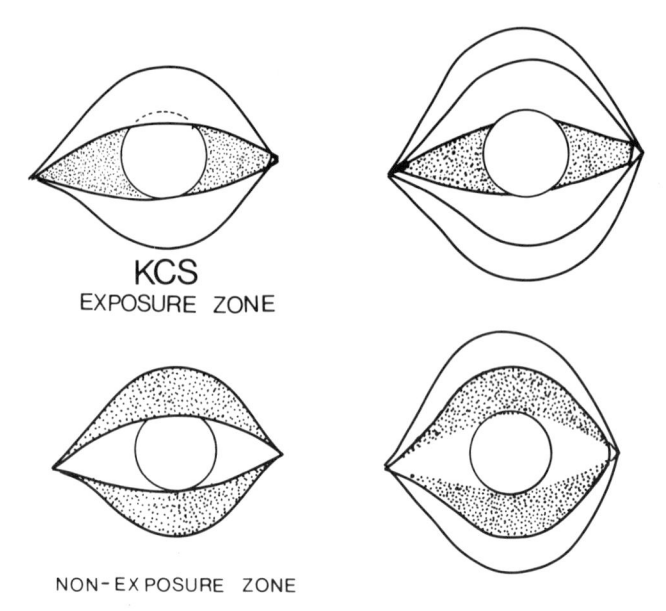

Figure 4 *The exposure zone and nonexposure zone (indicated by shaded area) of both normal (left panel) and forcefully opened (right panel) eye position. The exposure zone staining is characteristic for keratoconjunctivitis sicca (KCS).*

Patterns of Staining and Differential Diagnosis Although the intensity of rose bengal staining has been graded [54], the most valuable information with respect to diagnosis is the topographical pattern of the staining. Because unstable tear film invariably starts from the exposed area of ocular surface, the staining pattern characteristic of dry eyes should involve the exposure zone more than the nonexposure zone. The exposure and nonexposure zones are depicted respectively in the schematic drawing in Figure 4. Evaluation of positive dye staining without making note of the topographical distribution is not meaningful. Inasmuch as exposure zone staining is characteristic of dry eyes, the preferential nonexposure zone staining is characteristic of other non-dry-eye ocular surface disorders.

Grading Disease Severity Because the ocular surface change can develop after the primary abnormality in tear stability and protection, this change detected by dye stainings or impression cytology can be used as an index of disease severity. The milder form of dry eyes will reveal abnormalities in one or more tear functional tests without any dye staining. In contrast, the more severe form of dry eyes will invariably be accompanied by positive dye stainings. Furthermore, the severity of dry-eye conditions is parallel to the extent of positive dye stainings.

This investigation was supported in part by Public Health Service Research Grant #EY06819 (SCGT), Department of Health and Human Services, from the National Eye Institute, Bethesda, MD.

■ References

1. Holly FJ, Lemp MA. Tear physiology and dry eyes. Review. Surv Ophthalmol 1977; 22:69–87
2. Holly FJ. Basic factors underlying the formation and stability of the preocular tear film. In: Cavanagh HD, ed. The cornea: transactions of the World Congress on the Cornea III. New York: Raven Press, 1988:1–4
3. Duke-Elder S, ed. Physiology of the eye: vol 11, System of ophthalmology. London: Henry Kimpton, 1977:411–432
4. Allen A. Mucus—a protective secretion of complexity. TIBS 1983;5:169–173
5. Carlstedt I, Sheehan JK, Corfield AP, Gallagher JT. Mucous glycoproteins: a gel of a problem. Essays Biochem 1985;20:40–76
6. Iwata S. Fractionation and chemical properties of tear mucoids. Exp Eye Res 1971; 12:360–367
7. Moore JC, Tiffany JM. Human ocular mucus. Origins and preliminary characterization. Exp Eye Res 1979;29:291–301
8. Moore JC, Tiffany JM. Human ocular mucus. Chemical studies. Exp Eye Res 1981; 33:203–212
9. Chao CCW, Vergnes JP, Brown SI. O-glycosidic linkage in glycoprotein isolates from human ocular mucus. Exp Eye Res 1983;37:533–541
10. Chao CCW, Butala SM, Herp A. Studies on the isolation and composition of human ocular mucin. Exp Eye Res 1988;47:185–196
11. Tseng SCG, Huang AJW, Sutter D. Purification and characterization of rabbit ocular mucin. Invest Ophthalmol Vis Sci 1987;28:1473–1482
12. Wolff E. Anatomy of eye and orbit, ed 4. New York: Blakiston, 1954:207–209
13. Nichols B, Dawson CR, Togni B. Surface features of the conjunctiva and cornea. Invest Ophthalmol Vis Sci 1983;24:570–576
14. Nichols BA, Chiappino ML, Dawson CR. Demonstration of the mucous layer of the tear film by electron microscopy. Invest Ophthalmol Vis Sci 1985;26:464–473
15. Dilly PN. Contribution of the epithelium to the stability of the tear film. Trans Ophthalmol Soc UK 1985;104:381–389
16. Hazlett LD, Moon MM. Ocular surface complex carbohydrates are modified with aging. Exp Eye Res 1987;44:89–100
17. Watanabe H, Tisdale AS, Gipson IK. Eyelid opening induces expression of glycocalyx glycoprotein of rat ocular surface epithelium. Invest Ophthalmol Vis Sci 1993; 34:327–338
18. Adams AD. The morphology of human conjunctival mucus. Arch Ophthalmol 1979;97:730–734
19. Greiner JV, Weidman TA, Korb DR, Allansmith MR. Histochemical analysis of secretory vesicles in nongoblet conjunctival epithelial cells. Acta Ophthalmol (Copenh) 1985;63:8992
20. Wells PA, DeSiena-Shaw C, Rice B, Foster CS. Detection of ocular mucus in normal human conjunctiva and conjunctiva from patients with cicatricial pemphigoid using lectin probes and histochemical techniques. Exp Eye Res 1988;46:485–497
21. Kawano K, Uehara F, Ohba N. Lectin-cytochemical study on epithelial mucus glycoprotein of conjunctiva and pterygium. Exp Eye Res 1988;47:43–51

22. Huang AJW, Tseng SCG. Development of monocular antibodies to rabbit ocular mucin. Invest Ophthalmol Vis Sci 1987;28:1483–1491
23. Mui MM, Tseng SCG. Characterization or monoclonal antibodies against mucosal epithelium membrane-associated mucin-like protein (MEM). Invest Ophthalmol Vis Sci 1992;33(S):1176
24. Chang HA, Tseng SCG. Characterization of precorneal mucus layer. Invest Ophthalmol Vis Sci 1992;33(S):951
25. Sjögren H. Zur Kenntnis der Keratoconjunctivitis sicca (Keratitis filiformis bei hypofunktion der Tranendrusen). Acta Ophthalmol (Copenh) 1933;suppl 2
26. Passmore JW, King JH Jr. Vital staining of conjunctiva and cornea. Review of literature and critical study of certain dyes. Arch Ophthalmol 1955;53:568–574
27. Norn MS. Vital staining of cornea and conjunctiva. Acta Ophthalmol (Copenh) 1962;40:389–401
28. Norn MS. Dead, degenerate, and living cells in conjunctival fluid and mucous thread. Acta Ophthalmol (Copenh) 1969;47:1102–1115
29. Fox RI, Howell FV, Bone RC, Michelson P. Primary Sjögren syndrome: clinical and immunopathologic features. Semin Arthritis Rheum 1984;14:77–105
30. Marsh RJ, Fraunfelder FT, McGill JI. Herpetic corneal epithelial disease. Arch Ophthalmol 1976;94:1899–1902
31. Wilson FM II. Rose bengal staining of epibulbar squamous neoplasms. Ophthalmic Surg 1976;7:21–23
32. Pavan-Langston D, ed. Manual of ocular diagnosis and therapy, ed 2. Boston: Little, Brown, 1985:76–77
33. Huang AJW, Watson BD, Hernandez E, Tseng SCG. Photothrombosis of corneal neovascularization by intravenous rose bengal and argon laser irradiation. Arch Ophthalmol 1988;106:680–685
34. Feenstra RPG, Chen CF, Watson BD, Tseng SCG. Photodynamic effect of rose bengal on cultured cells. Invest Ophthalmol Vis Sci 1990;31(S):478
35. Feenstra RPG, Tseng SCG. What is actually stained by rose bengal? Arch Ophthalmol 1992;110:984–993
36. Feenstra RPG, Tseng SCG. Comparison of fluorescein and rose bengal staining. Ophthalmology 1992;99:605–617
37. Fullard RJ, Snyder C. Protein levels in nonstimulated and stimulated tears of normal human subjects. Invest Ophthalmol Vis Sci 1990;31(6):1119–1126
38. Zhang SH, Tseng SCG. Interactions between rose bengal (RB) and tear components. Invest Ophthalmol Vis Sci 1992;35(S):1286
39. Mishima S. Some physiological aspects of the precorneal tear film. Arch Ophthalmol 1965;73:233–241
40. Holly FJ, Lemp MA. Wettability and wetting of corneal epithelium. Exp Eye Res 1971;11:239–250
41. Lemp MA, Dohlman CH, Kuwabara T. Dry eye secondary to mucus deficiency. Trans Am Acad Ophthalmol Otolaryngol 1971;75:1223–1227
42. Dohlman CH, Friend J, Kalevar V, et al. The glycoprotein (mucus) content of tears from normals and dry eye patients. Exp Eye Res 1976;22:359–365
43. Holly FJ, Patten JT, Dohlman CH. Surface activity determination of aqueous tear components in dry eye patients and normals. Exp Eye Res 1977;24:479–491
44. Chodosh J, Banks MC, Stroop WG. Rose bengal inhibits herpes simplex virus replication in vero and human corneal epithelial cells in vitro. Invest Ophthalmol Vis Sci 1992;33:2520–2527
45. Eliason JA, Maurice DM. Staining of conjunctiva and conjunctival tear film. Br J Ophthalmol 1990;74:519–522
46. Norn MS. Lissamine green. Vital staining of cornea and conjunctiva. Acta Ophthalmol (Copenh) 1973;51:483–491

47. Emran N, Sommer A. Lissamine green staining in the clinical diagnosis of xerophthalmia. Arch Ophthalmol 1979;97:2333–2335
48. Nommensen FE, Dekkers NWHM. Detection of measles antigen in conjunctival epithelial lesions staining by lissamine green during measles virus infection. J Med Virol 1981;7:157–162
49. Mui MM, Tseng SCG. The lack of tear mucus protection as a possible mechanism for preferential antigen presentation in MALT. Invest Ophthalmol Vis Sci 1993; 34(s):1470
50. Chodosh J, Dix RD, Howell RC, et al. Staining characteristics and antiviral activity of sulforhodamine B and lissamine green B. Invest Ophthalmol Vis Sci 1993; 34(s):1470
51. Nelson JD, Havener VR, Cameron JD. Cellulose acetate impressions of the ocular surface; dry eye states. Arch Ophthalmol 1983;101:1869–1872
52. Tseng SCG. Staging of conjunctival squamous metaplasia by impression cytology. Ophthalmology 1985;92:728–733
53. Pflugfelder SC, Huang AJW, Schuchovski PT, et al. Cytological features of primary Sjögren syndrome. Ophthalmology 1990;97:985–991
54. van Bijsterveld OP. Diagnostic tests in the sicca syndrome. Arch Ophthalmol 1969; 82:10–14

Systemic Diseases Associated with Dry Eye

Robert I. Fox, M.D., Ph.D.

Dryness of the eye is a very common complaint, particularly among the elderly. It is important to determine clinically whether this dryness results from a local problem, requiring only symptomatic relief by artificial lubricants, or from a systemic disease process that requires further diagnostic tests and therapy. Systemic problems may include autoimmune disorders (such as primary and secondary Sjögren's syndrome), infiltrative disorders (such as lymphoma, amyloidosis, or hemachromatosis), and processes that affect the autonomic neural innervation of the gland (including medication side effects and diseases such as multiple sclerosis).

It is important for the ophthalmologist to be familiar with systemic illnesses associated with dry eyes because he or she may be the first physician to see these patients and must decide whether referral to other specialists and administration of systemic medications are required. In an era of prepaid medical insurance plans, i.e., health maintenance organizations (HMOs), the use of specific resources (including consultations and laboratory analysis) must be carefully considered. In addition, the presence of a systemic disease may greatly influence the types of problems that an ophthalmologist may encounter in a dry-eye patient, particularly during surgery and in the postoperative period.

The current body of literature about the systemic manifestations of dry eye is very confusing. This has become most apparent in the controversy over the definition of Sjögren's syndrome, for which there are no universally accepted criteria for diagnosis. The ophthalmologist needs to be knowledgeable about this controversy to help counsel the patient about the prognosis and specific therapy.

■ Primary Sjögren's Syndrome

Background

The most common autoimmune disease associated with ocular dryness is Sjögren's syndrome (SS), a condition including keratoconjunctivitis sicca

(KCS) in association with xerostomia. SS patients have symptoms of dryness of the eyes (generally described as a gritty sensation) and the mouth (difficulty eating a dry cracker without water). They may have swollen major salivary glands (i.e., parotid and submandibular) and cervical lymphadenopathy. The condition was originally called *Mikulicz's disease,* in reference to dryness associated with lymphocytic infiltrates of glands. However, this term was used to describe such a wide spectrum of diseases (including lymphoma, sarcoidosis, and tuberculosis) that it currently lacks either diagnostic or prognostic specificity. In 1932, Henrik Sjögren described the association of KCS and rheumatoid arthritis. The syndrome was rediscovered by Morgan and Castleman in 1953 [1] and described in more detail by Bloch and coworkers in 1956 [2]. Although there is general agreement on the ocular component of SS (i.e., KCS), there is no agreement on how to define the oral component (xerostomia), which has resulted in confusion in clinical practice and in the research literature. The problem of diagnostic criteria is reviewed in this chapter and in more detail in a recent issue of the *Rheumatic Disease Clinics of North America* [3].

Depending on the classification system used, the incidence of SS will vary almost 100-fold, ranging from 0.1% (using either the San Francisco or San Diego criteria) to 5% of the entire population (using certain European criteria). As in other autoimmune diseases, there is a marked (90%) predominance among women. Using the San Diego criteria, there are two peak ages of onset. A younger group of patients (age 20 to 40 years) frequently has onset of dry eyes and systemic manifestations similar to patients with systemic lupus erythematosus (SLE). In a second group of patients, onset occurs at age 60 or older, and this group generally has fewer systemic manifestations. This older group closely overlaps with the elderly population with lupus. In addition, SS can occur in children as part of the spectrum of juvenile rheumatoid arthritides.

Different Methods for Classification of SS

The diagnostic criteria for SS remain unclear because there is no international agreement on classification, which had led to confusion in clinical practice and in the research literature. Indeed, it is likely that much of the controversy over the association of SS with other disorders (including lymphoma, dementia, and multiple sclerosis–like illnesses) and the response to specific therapies derives in large part from the different types of SS patients enrolled at different medical centers. Three types of classification criteria are widely used: the San Francisco criteria, the San Diego criteria, and the European criteria.

The San Francisco Criteria Patients fulfilling the San Francisco classification criteria [4] have KCS plus a characteristic minor salivary gland biopsy. Figure 1A shows the lymphocytic infiltrates in a SS biopsy com-

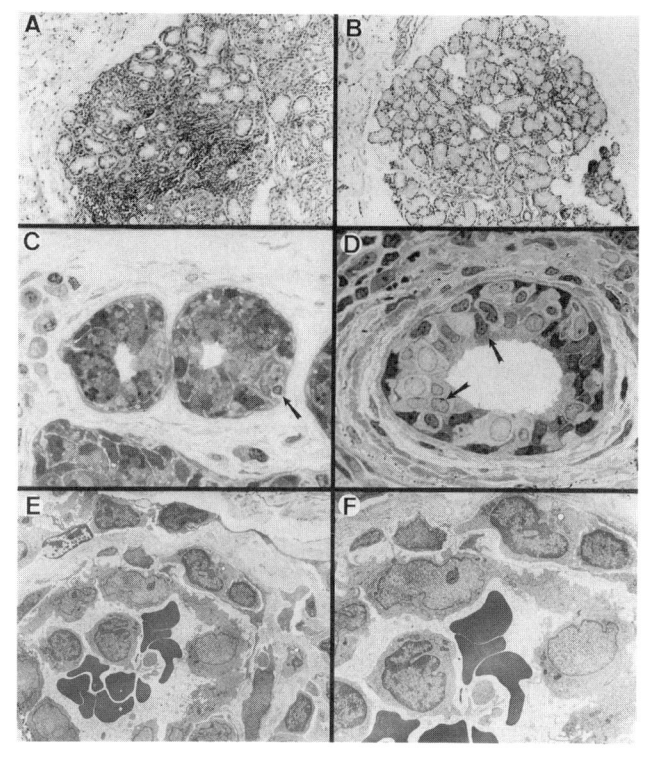

Figure 1 *Minor salivary gland biopsies from normals and patients with Sjögren's syndrome. (A) In a patient with Sjögren's syndrome, a focal lymphocytic infiltrate is present in the center portion of the lobule. (B) Biopsy specimen obtained at autopsy from an individual lacking evidence of any systemic autoimmune disease. (C, D) Higher-magnification views of lymphocytes (arrows) infiltrating acinar and ductal cells in a Sjögren's syndrome patient. (E, F) Higher-magnification views (taken with electron microscope) of high endothelial venules in a Sjögren's syndrome patient.*

pared to a normal salivary gland biopsy (see Fig 1B). The key feature of the SS biopsy is the presence of clusters (foci) of lymphocytes in an arrangement called *focal sialadenitis*. Each lymphocyte focus contains at least 50 (and often hundreds of) lymphocytes that are adjacent to relatively intact acini, ducts, or vascular endothelial cells. The number of foci per 4 mm^2 is determined, and a high correlation with KCS exists when the average focus score (based on at least four evaluable glands) is greater than 1. Important sources of error are failure to determine the average focus score, and simply to report the number of foci in a single lobule and failure to exclude lobules where ductal ectasia and rupture lead to a nonspecific inflammatory infiltrate.

The minor salivary gland biopsy with focal sialadenitis has a high degree of correlation with the presence of autoantibodies. In comparison, minor salivary gland biopsies with scattered lymphocytic infiltrates are nonspecific and *not* closely associated with autoantibodies. An additional source of confusion is that multiple different scoring systems are used to report the results of salivary gland biopsies, and the physician must be certain that the pathologist is using the currently accepted system. In particular, the older systems of Chisholm and Mason [5] and Tarpley [6] do not adequately distinguish focal sialadenitis from chronic nonspecific sialadenitis and thus are not sufficiently sensitive to be useful for diagnosing SS.

The San Diego Criteria The San Diego classification system [7] uses a combination of clinical and laboratory criteria (Table 1). Patients should have objective evidence of dry eyes and dry mouth. Further, they should exhibit evidence of a systemic autoimmune process in the form of autoantibodies such as antinuclear antibody (titer $> 1:320$) or rheumatoid factor (anti-IgG Fc, titer $> 1:320$). The antinuclear antibody often has a fine speckled pattern owing to the occurrence of antibodies against ribonuclear antigens, termed *SS-A* (Sjögren's-associated A) or *SS-B* antigen, alternately known as *Ro* and *La*, respectively. The absence of these autoantibodies makes us search harder for other processes—including lymphoma, sarcoidosis, or infections such as retrovirus—that may cause increasing dry-

Table 1 *San Diego Criteria for Sjögren's Syndrome*

I. Primary Sjögren's syndrome (SS)*
   A. Symptoms and objective signs of ocular dryness
      1. Schirmer's test less than 8 mm wetting per 5 minutes *and*
      2. Positive rose bengal or fluorescein staining of cornea *or* conjunctiva to demonstrate keratoconjunctivitis sicca
   B. Symptoms and objective signs of dry mouth
      1. Decreased parotid flow rate using Lashley cups or other methods *and*
      2. Abnormal biopsy of minor salivary gland (focus score of ≥ 2 based on average of 4 evaluable lobules)
   C. Evidence of a systemic autoimmune disorder
      1. Elevated rheumatoid factor $\geq 1:320$ *or*
      2. Elevated antinuclear antibody $\geq 1:320$ *or*
      3. Presence of anti-SS-A (Ro) or anti-SS-B (La) antibodies
II. Secondary Sjögren's syndrome: characteristic signs and symptoms of SS (described in I) plus clinical features sufficient to allow a diagnosis of rheumatoid arthritis, systemic lupus erythematosus, polymyositis, scleroderma, or biliary cirrhosis
III. Exclusions: sarcoidosis, preexistent lymphoma, acquired immunodeficiency disease, and other known causes of keratitis sicca or salivary gland enlargement

*Definite Sjögren's syndrome requires objective evidence of dryness of eyes and mouth and a systemic autoimmune process, including a characteristic minor salivary gland biopsy. *Probable* Sjögren's syndrome does not require a minor salivary gland biopsy but can be diagnosed with demonstration of decreased salivary function (I.B.1).

ness. In patients who lack features of a systemic autoimmune process (i.e., absent autoantibodies and absent acute-phase reactants) but who have significant dryness, we assign the diagnosis of sicca syndrome or dry eye rather than SS.

Copenhagen Criteria and European Cooperative Study Group The European classification criteria [8, 9] are dependent on clinical observations and do not require evaluation of biopsy or autoantibodies. For example, a patient with KCS and diminished salivary gland flow can receive a diagnosis of SS. As discussed by Daniels [4], this definition of *xerostomia* is sufficiently vague that it does not adequately distinguish among patients with focal sialadenitis, chronic sialadenitis, and even normal lip biopsies. As a result, a much higher proportion of the general population (up to 5% of adults older than 50 years) would be classified as having SS by the European criteria, in comparison to fewer than 1% using the San Diego or San Francisco criteria. When a group of patients labeled as having SS by the European criteria was reassessed using the San Diego criteria, only 22% of the group was considered to have SS. Advocates of the European criteria believe that the more restrictive San Diego criteria identify only the tip of the iceberg. In contrast, I believe that restrictive criteria (i.e., the San Diego criteria) are helpful in research studies to identify a subgroup that may share a common etiopathogenesis.

Extraglandular Manifestations in the SS Patient

In patients with primary SS, a wide spectrum of extraglandular manifestations may be present, including skin rashes such as leukocytoclastic vasculitis and hypergammaglobulinemic purpura. These patients may have lung symptoms including pleurisy and interstitial pneumonitis. They can develop interstitial nephritis and a wide spectrum of central nervous system symptoms. In general, all the systemic manifestations associated with SLE can also occur in primary SS patients, although there are minor differences between them (i.e., interstitial nephritis rather than glomerulonephritis; increased risk of lymphoproliferative diseases).

Differential Diagnosis of Symptoms of Dryness

Salivary and tear flow varies widely in normal individuals and factors including age, sex, diet, smoking, depression, and anxiety can strongly influence the frequency of sicca symptoms. It is important to reassure patients who lack evidence of a significant autoimmune disease that they have a local problem which can be treated by conservative measures (artificial lubricants, punctal occlusion, etc.) and that they do not have a progressive systemic disorder [10]. The advent of patient newsletters and patient support groups for dry-eye patients, as well as articles about Sjögren's syndrome that appear in the lay press, has led to disproportionate anxiety and overtreatment of some normal individuals.

Symptoms of eye dryness may be mimicked by local eye irritation (blepharitis), nutritional deficiencies (vitamin A), allergic reactions (Stevens-Johnson syndrome), infections (trachoma), neoplastic disorders that infiltrate the gland (especially lymphomas), and prior radiation therapy to the head. Enlargement of the salivary glands or lacrimal glands may reflect an infiltrative process such as lymphoma, sarcoidosis, amyloidosis, hemachromatosis, or fatty infiltrates found in patients with elevated cholesterol, excess alcohol consumption, and diabetes.

■ Secondary Sjögren's Syndrome

SS Associated with Rheumatoid Arthritis

Rheumatoid arthritis (RA) is the most common autoimmune disorder associated with dry eyes and may affect up to 1% of the general population. Up to 20% of patients with severe RA may develop KCS. Usually, the sicca symptoms in RA patients occur many years after the onset of joint symptoms. However, some patients may have early onset of sicca symptoms and limited joint swelling, particularly patients with Felty's syndrome. Rheumatoid nodules, generally located over extensor tendons such as the elbows, are associated with increased arthritis severity, increased frequency of extraarticular manifestation of RA, including ocular manifestations such as KCS, nodular scleritis, and corneal vasculitis (corneal melting). Ironically, KCS and corneal vasculitis can occur in the late-stage RA patient in whom the joint symptoms are relatively quiescent.

Clinical features associated with RA include symmetrical involvement of the wrists and proximal finger joints (such as the metacarpal and proximal interphalangeal joints) (Fig 2). Other joints, among them knees and feet, are also involved but are less obvious for evaluation by the ophthalmologist. In contrast to the proximal finger involvement due to RA, osteoarthritis generally spares these proximal joints and affects the distal finger

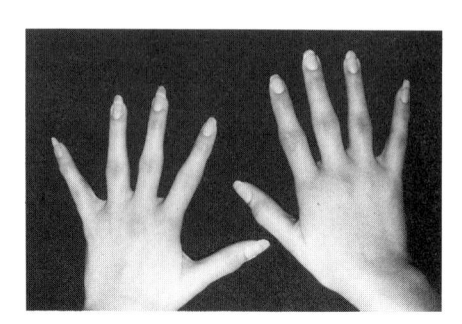

Figure 2 *Swelling of the proximal interphalangeal joints in a patient with early rheumatoid arthritis.*

joints (i.e., the distal interphalangeal). Another hint that RA is present is a high rheumatoid factor in the patient's serum; this autoantibody is directed against the Fc region of the IgG molecule and generally is reported as a titer measured by the latex agglutination method and, more recently, by enzyme-linked immunosorbent assay methods.

In some RA patients, the rheumatoid factor test is negative and the clinical diagnosis is confirmed by the characteristic radiographic appearance of joint erosions. Important subgroups of seronegative patients include psoriatic arthritis, Reiter's syndrome, juvenile polyarthritis (including onset in adulthood) and Lyme arthritis. Asymmetrical (and particularly monoarticular) arthritis is more frequent in rheumatoid factor–negative patients.

The sudden onset of monoarticular joint swelling in any patient should suggest an infectious or crystalline (i.e., gout or pseudogout) cause. Joint aspiration for culture is usually required for differential diagnosis. Failure to treat an infected joint promptly can lead to rapid destruction of the affected joint and associated septicemia.

SS Associated with SLE

Many of the clinical features found in primary SS patients—including arthralgias, myalgias, pleurisy, pericarditis, and central nervous system manifestations—are also found in SLE patients. The presence of a malar rash (i.e., a macular rash over the nose and cheeks but sparing the nasolabial fold; Fig 3) is a frequent clue to coexistent SLE in the dry-eye patient. It is now recognized that SLE is a heterogeneous group of diseases, with one clinical subset of patients exhibiting glomerulonephritis and a distinct subset with KCS [11]. The SLE subset with secondary SS shares a common genetic predisposition (i.e., HLA-DR3) and autoantibodies (antinuclear antibody, SS-A, SS-B) with primary SS patients [12], which suggests a common etiopathogenesis of an SLE subset and primary SS [13].

The sicca symptoms associated with SLE occur first at two distinct age intervals. Onset may occur when the patient is between 20 and 30 years old; a second peak occurs after age 50 years. These patterns of onset parallel the findings in primary SS patients (San Diego criteria). Thus, the clinical distinction between primary and secondary SS associated with SLE may be very difficult and generally is based on characteristic laboratory abnormalities.

The differential diagnosis of ocular pain in the SLE patient with secondary SS often is challenging, particularly when the patient is on highly immunosuppressive medications. Bacterial, viral, and fungal infections must be considered. Also consideration of orbital vasculitis (Fig 4) is important when ocular symptoms are out of proportion to the objective findings of KCS.

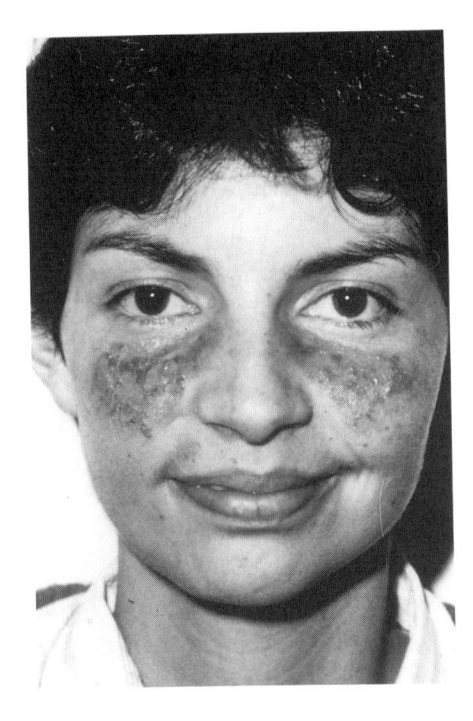

Figure 3 Malar rash in a patient with systemic lupus erythematosus.

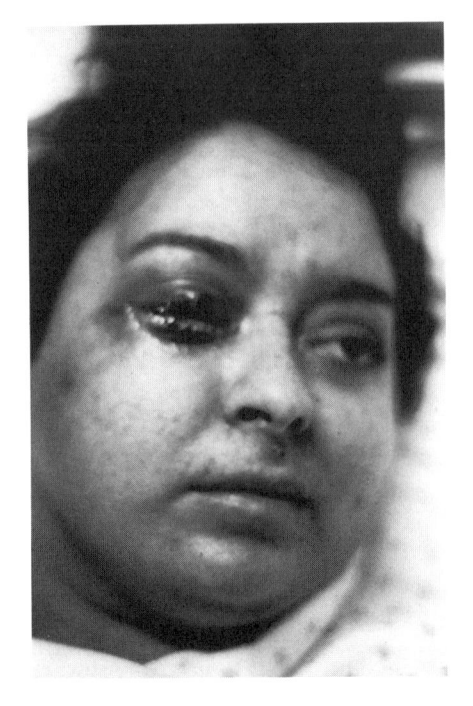

Figure 4 Orbital vasculitis in a patient with Sjögren's syndrome. Complaints of increased periorbital pain resulted from a vasculitic infarct.

SS Associated with Progressive Systemic Sclerosis

Progressive systemic sclerosis (PSS, or scleroderma) is characterized by thickening of the skin. Clues to the diagnosis of PSS is a history of Raynaud's phenomenon and the observation of telangiectasias in the nail beds, as these signs may precede the development of overt sclerodermatous skin changes. PSS patients often have a positive antinuclear antibody test, with an anticentromere or antinucleolar pattern.

At least two subgroups of PSS patients are currently recognized that differ in their clinical onset and prognosis. Patients with limited PSS have skin tightening distal to their elbows and knees; included in this group are patients previously given a diagnosis of *CREST* (calcinosis, Raynaud's phenomenon, esophageal dysfunction, sclerodactyly, and telangiectasia). Patients with diffuse PSS have both skin manifestations proximal to the elbows and knees and a higher incidence of visceral involvement, including renal involvement. In both groups, the minor salivary gland biopsies may show fibrosis rather than lymphocytic infiltrates. The limited PSS patients usually have antibodies against the centromere owing to their reaction against centromere-associated proteins cenp-A and cenp-B, whereas diffuse PSS patients have antibodies against topoisomerase, an antigen previously termed *Scl-70*.

SS Associated with Dermatomyositis and Primary Biliary Cirrhosis

The occurrence of severe muscle pains and a facial rash with a purple heliotrope on the upper eyelids should suggest the diagnosis of dermatomyositis. This diagnosis is confirmed by elevation of muscle enzymes (creatine phosphokinase and aldolase). In the absence of characteristic skin rash, the condition is termed *polymyositis*.

Biliary cirrhosis is an autoimmune disorder characterized by lymphocytic infiltrates in the portal triad of the liver. These patients frequently have a positive antinuclear antibody test and a characteristic antibody against the mitochondrial enzyme 2-oxaloacetic acid/dehydrogenase [14]. They are distinguished from primary SS patients by their elevated liver function tests and their autoantibody profile.

■ Differential Diagnosis of SS

Infiltrative Diseases

Any process that replaces the lacrimal and salivary gland tissues, such as lymphoma, hemochromatosis, and amyloidosis, soon results in dryness (Table 2). In addition, glandular swelling can result from the deposition

Table 2 *Systemic Diseases and Laboratory Abnormalities Associated with Dry Eye*

   I. Autoimmune disorders
      A. Primary Sjögren's syndrome
         1. Abnormal labial salivary gland biopsy (focal sialadenitis)
         2. Antinuclear antibody (ANA) with fine speckled pattern
         3. Antibody against SS-A (Ro) and SS-B (La) ribonuclear proteins
      B. Secondary Sjögren's syndrome associated with:
         1. Rheumatoid arthritis
         2. Systemic lupus erythematosus
         3. Progressive systemic sclerosis (scleroderma)
         4. Polymyositis and dermatomyositis
         5. Primary biliary cirrhosis
      C. Graft-versus-host disease
      D. Immune reactions after radiation to head and neck
  II. Infiltrative process
      A. Lymphoma
      B. Amyloidosis
      C. Hemochromatosis
      D. Sarcoidosis (Hereford's syndrome)
 III. Infectious processes
      A. HIV-diffuse infiltrative lymphadenopathy syndrome (DILS)
      B. Hepatitis B and hepatitis C
      C. Syphilis
      D. Trachoma
      E. Tuberculosis
  IV. Neuropathic dysfunction of the glands
      A. Multiple sclerosis
      B. Cranial neuropathies (seventh nerve)
         1. Bell's palsy
         2. Vasculitis

HIV = human immunodeficiency virus.

of fat in the glands associated with diabetes, alcoholism, pancreatitis, cirrhosis, and hypertriglyceridemia.

Infectious Diseases

Several infectious processes can mimic SS (see Table 2). Historically, both tuberculosis and syphilis can cause infiltrative lesions that replace glandular tissue. In certain areas of the world and in patients with increasing immunosuppression, consideration of these possibilities is necessary.

Sicca symptoms can develop in patients with retroviral infections due to human T-lymphotropic virus type 1 (HTLV-1) (particularly in endemic areas) and in individuals infected with the human immunodeficiency virus (HIV). A condition called the *diffuse infiltrative lymphadenopathy syndrome* (DILS) occurs in HIV-infected patients [14]. It is more common in children (up to 10% of neonatal HIV cases) and occurs in approximately 0.5% of HIV-infected adults. Recognition of this syndrome is important for reasons of both safety (correct disposal of infected materials for protection of health care professionals) and early therapy using antiviral medications. DILS patients differ from SS patients in the types of lymphocytes that infiltrate their salivary gland biopsies (i.e., a predominance of CD8+ T cells) [15] and in the absence of antibodies to nuclear antigens.

Patients with hepatitis C infection may develop autoimmune features including sicca symptoms and mixed cryoglobulinemia. Again, prompt recognition of these patients is important for both patient care and correct disposal of hazardous materials.

Side Effects of Medications

Anticholinergic side effects occur in patients receiving a wide spectrum of medications for blood pressure, depression, and cardiac arrhythmia (Table 3). Frequently, older patients with mild sicca symptoms will experience significant exacerbation of these symptoms due to these medications. Significant improvement may be achieved simply by using alternative drugs that lack these side effects.

Table 3 *Medications with Anticholinergic Side Effects*

Blood pressure
   Clonidine and prazosin (alpha$_1$-blocker)
   Prazosin (Minipress) (alpha$_2$-blocker)
   Propranolol (Inderal) (beta blocker)
   Reserpine
   Methyldopa (Aldomet) and guanethidine
Antidepressants (tricyclics and monoamine oxidase inhibitors)
   Amitriptyline (Elavil) and nortriptyline (Pamelor)
   Imipramine (Tofranil) and desipramine (Norpramin)
   Doxepin (Sinequan)
   Phenelzine (Nardil) and tranylcypromine (Parnate)
   Amoxapine (Asendin) and trimipramine (Surmontil)
Cardiac antiarrhythmic drugs
   Disopyramide (Norpace)
   Mexiletine
Parkinson's disease (anticholinergic agents)
   Trihexyphenidyl
   Benztropine
   Biperiden
   Procyclidine
Antiulcer agents
   Atropine-like drugs
   Metoclopramide (Reglan) and other drugs that decrease gastric motility
Muscle spasms
   Cyclobenzaprine (Flexeril)
   Methocarbamol (Robaxin)
Decongestants (over-the-counter cold remedies)
   Ephedrine
   Pseudoephedrine

Other Conditions Associated with Dryness

Graft-versus-host disease (GVHD) after bone marrow transplantation results in lymphocytic infiltration and a sicca syndrome. Presumably, immune responses against the foreign histocompatibility antigens play an important role in this disease's pathogenesis. Although initially considered to be similar to SS, GVHD has been found, in subsequent studies of biopsy specimens, to bear a closer similarity to severe lichen planus [16].

Progressive dryness can develop in patients who have had radiation to the head and neck. This process may develop years after the initial radiation and may represent an induced form of autoimmune reaction against antigens liberated from the damaged tissue.

Sarcoidosis may present with glandular swelling and sicca symptoms, although anterior uveitis is a more common ocular manifestation. The presence of noncaseating granulomatous infiltrates, elevated angiotensin-converting enzyme (ACE), and an abnormal chest radiograph (hilar adenopathy) help distinguish sarcoidosis from SS.

Patients with multiple sclerosis have problems with dry eyes and dry mouth, probably due to interference with the cholinergic innervation of their glands. However, a subset of SS patients exhibit multiple sclerosis–like symptoms and abnormal brain scans on magnetic resonance imaging due to focal lymphocytic infiltrates in their brains.

Blepharitis and blepharospasm can mimic or exacerbate dry-eye symptoms. Blepharitis results from blockage or infection of the meibomian glands. Increased symptoms in a Sjögren's patient in whom KCS appears to have improved on examination by rose bengal (or fluorescein) staining should suggest this possibility. Blepharitis frequently occurs in SS patients who are using excessive amounts of ocular lubricant at night (thereby blocking the gland) and is sometimes exacerbated by artificial tears that contain preservatives. The use of eyelid scrubs, temporary avoidance of lubricating gels, and the switch to a preservative-free tear solution may prove helpful.

Blepharospasm, a condition characterized by uncontrollable blinking, may result from damage to a particular nerve plexus controlling the blink reflex. Sicca symptoms may contribute to the patient's discomfort, but the symptoms and a blink rate in excess of the objective findings of KCS suggest this problem. The recent introduction of botulinum toxin injections for this problem may be helpful.

■ Pathogenesis of SS

Essential features of SS (as defined by San Francisco or San Diego criteria) include focal lymphoid infiltrates in the lacrimal and salivary glands and the presence of autoantibodies. Under higher magnification (see Fig 1C, 1D), lymphocytes can be seen in direct contact with glandular epithelial cells. Immunohistological studies indicate that these are predominantly CD4+ T cells [17] with Tαβ antigen receptor and memory phenotype [18] that exhibit helper T-cell function [19]. Another important feature of the SS salivary gland biopsy is the expression of HLA-DR (i.e., major histocompatibility complex class II) antigens on the glandular epithelial cells, in contrast to normal glandular epithelial cells, which lack HLA-DR expression [20, 21]. The presence of cell surface HLA-DR allows these epithelial cells to present exogenous and autoantigens to the CD4+ T cells [22]. Additional important features of the salivary gland biopsy include the conversion of capillaries to "high endothelial venules," structures that promote the migration of lymphocytes from the circulation into the gland (see Fig 1E). Also, higher magnification electron microscopic views of the basement membrane surrounding the blood vessels (see Fig 1F) do not show the electron dense deposits, i.e., the absence of immune complex deposition. Taken together, these features emphasize the importance of cell-mediated glandular destruction, rather than antibody or immune complex-complement mediated mechanisms.

A minority of the infiltrating salivary gland lymphocytes are B cells that can be stimulated to produce autoantibodies in vitro [19]. These B cells demonstrate preferential use of certain variable regions (especially the V-kappa III subgroup) [23, 24] and may exhibit oligoclonal expansion detected by Southern blot methods [25, 26]. Also, the vast majority of lymphomas that arise in SS patients are IgM-K B cells [27]. It seems that continued stimulation of the B cells by autoantigens or T-cell-derived factors leads to increased risk of lymphoma [28], perhaps due to karyotypical alterations induced by nucleases required for cell division, somatic diversification of antibody variable region segments, and isotype switching.

The actual mechanism of glandular destruction by the CD4+ T cells remains unknown but may involve induction of granzyme A and perforin [29]. These serine proteases are closely associated with lytic capacity of both CD4+ and CD8+ lymphocytes. It is unlikely that complement-mediated epithelial cell lysis (i.e., antibody plus complement) [30] or natural killer cells [19, 31] play a primary role in glandular destruction.

A variety of cytokines are produced within the salivary gland. Interleukin 2 (IL2), interferon gamma (IFN-γ), tumor necrosis factor–alpha (TNFα), and IL10 are produced by the salivary gland epithelial cells (Kang and associates, unpublished data, 1993). IFN-γ appears to play a key role in HLA-DR induction in salivary gland epithelial cells [20], as this induction is blocked by monoclonal antibodies to IFN-γ. IL6 and IL10 in synergistic interaction with other cytokines may promote B-cell growth and failure of tolerance mechanisms, may prevent apoptosis (i.e., preprogrammed cell death), and may be important factors in both autoimmunity and lymphoproliferation [32–34].

Although lymphocytic infiltration and destruction of salivary gland epithelial cells are important in decreased glandular function, it is likely that neuroendocrine factors also contribute to decreased glandular function [35]. Biopsy of the gland (see Fig 1A) shows that a significant proportion of acini and ducts at the edge of the lobule remain relatively intact. In comparison, kidneys and liver continue to secrete their characteristic products until more than 95% are destroyed; this residual glandular tissue can be seen in patients with profound dryness. It is likely that inflammatory cytokines (such as IL1 and TNF-α), released as a consequence of the inflammatory process, interfere with the neurogenic innervation of the remaining tissue. In a similar manner, a patient with the early stages of SS may be pushed into clinically overt dryness by the use of medications with anticholinergic activity or by emotional distress (i.e., anxiety or depression) that stimulates anticholinergic activity.

■ Special Therapeutic Considerations in the Dry-Eye Patient

Anesthesia and Surgery

Dry-eye patients are at increased risk of developing corneal abrasions intraoperatively and in the postoperative setting. The low humidity of the operating room and the decreased blink reflex of the patient under anesthesia contribute to this problem. Administration of ocular lubricants preoperatively and in the postoperative recovery suite will minimize this risk.

Upper-airway dryness of the SS patient leads to the increased chance of mucous plug inspissation during the postoperative period, followed by obstructive pneumonias. The use of humidified oxygen and avoidance of medications that excessively dry the upper airways (i.e., those agents employed with anesthesia to control secretions) will help prevent this problem. Also adequate preoperative hydration and respiratory therapy to keep airways clear may be important.

In the standard preoperative and postoperative period, the patient is denied liquids. Under these conditions, the SS patient will have greatly increased oral problems owing to his or her inability to moisten the mouth by saliva secretion. The use of artificial saliva sprays both before and after surgery will greatly improve patient comfort.

In RA patients with secondary SS, consideration of arthritic involvement of the neck (especially at the C1–C2 level) may be important. Attempts to hyperextend the neck to intubate the patient may result in transection of the cervical spinal cord and paraplegia. When cervical involvement due to RA is suspected, extreme caution during nasotracheal intubation must be exercised, and often the patient is intubated in a soft cervical collar to avoid this problem.

The poor state of a Sjögren's patient's teeth presents a higher risk of damage to teeth during intubation. The anesthesiologist must be careful to avoid such damage, which can lead to loss of teeth and their subsequent aspiration. In addition, these patients will incur great expense in obtaining dentures to their remaining teeth should any tooth loss occur.

In many surgical procedures, antibiotics are given routinely. The patient with sicca symptoms is at increased risk for associated oral candidiasis, and so the use of topical oral antifungal drugs such as nystatin to help prevent this complication is recommended.

Precautions regarding steroid coverage are important because such patients may remain relatively partially adrenal-insufficient, even after an extended period off glucocorticoids. During the stress of surgery, hypotensive complications may occur if adequate steroid replacement is not provided. Many SS patients are receiving glucocorticoids (steroids) at the time of surgery or have received them in the 6-month interval prior to surgery.

Finally, assessment of the fluid status of the SS patient in the postoperative period may be relatively difficult. Normal clinical clues of adequate fluid status, such as the moisture in the ocular and oral membranes, may be misleading. Furthermore, some SS patients have interstitial nephritis, which prevents adequate urine concentration and fluid balance. This problem may be exacerbated by antibiotics such as aminoglycosides.

This clinical research program is supported by grants from the National Institutes of Health (MO1RR00833) and postdoctoral fellowships from the Price, Scripps, Hennings Ramsdell, and Thornton Charitable Foundations for Drs. Pavel and Eva Pisa, Hoil Kang, and Ichiro Saito.

I gratefully acknowledge the useful suggestions of Drs. M. Friedlaender (ophthalmology), J. Willems (gynecology), G. Izuno (dermatology), R. Simon (allergy), R. Stewart (oral medicine), L. Gannon (rheumatology), and B. Towle (immunology).

■ References

1. Morgan W, Castleman B. A clinicopathologic study of Mikulicz's disease. Am J Pathol 1953;29:471–503
2. Bloch KJ, Buchanan WW, Wohl MJ, Bunim JJ. Sjögren's syndrome: a clinical, pathological and serological study of 62 cases. Medicine (Baltimore) 1956;44: 187–231
3. Fox R. Pathogenesis of Sjögren's syndrome. Rheum Dis Clin North Am 1993;18: 517–537
4. Daniels TE. Labial salivary gland biopsy in Sjögren's syndrome. Arthritis Rheum 1984;27:147–156
5. Chisholm DM, Mason DK. Labial salivary gland biopsy in Sjögren's disease. J Clin Pathol 1968;21:656–660
6. Tarpley T, Anderson L, White C. Minor salivary gland involvement in Sjögren's syndrome. Oral Surg 1974;37:64–73
7. Fox RI, Robinson CA, Curd JC, et al. Sjögren's syndrome: proposed criteria for classification. Arthritis Rheum 1986;29:577–585

8. Manthorpe R, Oxholm P, Prause JU, Schiödt M. The Copenhagen criteria for Sjögren's syndrome. Scand J Rheumatol Suppl 1986;61:19–21
9. Vitali C, Bombardieri S, Moutsopoulos HM, et al. Preliminary criteria for the classification of Sjögren's syndrome. Arthritis Rheum 1993;36:340–347
10. Lemp MA. Lacrimal hyposecretions. In: Fraunfelder FT, Roy FH, eds. Current ocular therapy, vol 2. Philadelphia: Saunders, 1985
11. Harley JB, Alexander EL, Bias WB, et al. Anti-Ro (SS-A) and Anti-La (SS-B) in patients with Sjögren's syndrome. Arthritis Rheum 1986;29:196–206
12. Manthorpe R, Teppo A, Bendixon G, Wegelius O. Antibodies to SS-B in chronic inflammatory connective tissue diseases. Relationship of HLA-Dw2 and HLA-Dw3 antigens in primary Sjögren's syndrome. Arthritis Rheum 1982;25:662–667
13. Kang H-I, Fei HM, Saito I, et al. Comparison of HLA class II genes in Caucasoid, Chinese, and Japanese patients with primary Sjögren's syndrome. J Immunol 1993; 150:3615–3623
14. Itescu S. Diffuse infiltrative lymphocytosis syndrome in human immunodeficiency virus infection—a Sjögren's-like disease. Rheum Dis Clin North Am 1991;17: 99–115
15. Itescu S, Brancato LJ, Buxbaum J, et al. A diffuse infiltrative CD8 lymphocytosis syndrome in human immunodeficiency virus (HIV) infection: a host immune response associated with HLA-DR5. Ann Intern Med 1990;112:3–10
16. Gratwhol AA, Moutsopoulos HM, Chused TM, et al. Sjögren-type syndrome after allogeneic bone-marrow transplantation. Ann Intern Med 1977;87:703–706
17. Adamson TC III, Fox RI, Frisman DM, Howell FV. Immunohistologic analysis of lymphoid infiltrates in primary Sjögren's syndrome using monoclonal antibodies. J Immunol 1983;130:203–208
18. Skopouli FN, Fox PC, Galanopoulou V, et al. T cell subpopulations in the labial minor salivary gland histopathologic lesion of Sjögren's syndrome. J Rheumatol 1991;18:210
19. Fox RI, Adamson TC III, Fong S, et al. Lymphocyte phenotype and function of pseudolymphomas associated with Sjögren's syndrome. J Clin Invest 1983;72: 52–62
20. Fox RI, Bumol T, Fantozzi R, et al. Expression of histocompatibility antigen HLA-DR by salivary gland epithelial cells in Sjögren's syndrome. Arthritis Rheum 1986; 29:1105–1111
21. Lindahl G, Hedfors E, Kloreskog L, Forsum U. Epithelial HLA-DR expression and T-cell subsets in salivary glands in Sjögren's syndrome. Clin Exp Immunol 1985;61:475–482
22. Unanue E. Antigen-presenting function of the macrophage. Annu Rev Immunol 1984;2:395–428
23. Fox RI, Carson DA, Chen P, Fong S. Characterization of a cross reactive idiotype in Sjögren's syndrome. Scand J Rheumatol 1986;561:83–88
24. Kipps TJ, Tomhave E, Chen PP, Fox RI. Molecular characterization of a major autoantibody-associated cross-reactive idiotype in Sjögren's syndrome. J Immunol 1989;142:4261–4268
25. Fishleder A, Tubbs R, Hesse B, Levin H. Immunoglobulin-gene rearrangement in benign lymphoepithelial lesions. N Engl J Med 1987;316:1118–1121
26. Freimark B, Fantozzi R, Bone R, et al. Detection of clonally expanded salivary gland lymphocytes in Sjögren's syndrome. Arthritis Rheum 1989;32:859–869
27. Schmid U, Helbron D, Lennert K. Development of malignant lymphoma in myoepithelial sialadenitis (Sjögren's syndrome). Virchows Arch 1982;395:11–41
28. Berard CW, Greene MH, Jaffe ES, et al. A multidisciplinary approach to non-Hodgkin's lymphoma: NIH conference. Ann Intern Med 1981;94:218–235
29. Griffiths GM, Alpert S, Su R, Weissman, I. The granzyme A gene: a marker for

cytolytic lymphocytes in vivo. In: Sitkovsky MV, Henkart PA, eds. Cytotoxic cells: regulation, effector function, generation and methods. Boston; 1993
30. MacSween RNM, Goudie RB, Anderson JR, et al. Occurrence of antibody to salivary duct epithelium in Sjögren's disease, rheumatoid arthritis, and other arthritides. Ann Rheum Dis 1967;26:402–410
31. Fox RI, Hugli TE, Lanier LL, et al. Salivary gland lymphocytes in primary Sjögren's syndrome lack lymphocyte subsets defined by Leu 7 and Leu 11 antigens. J Immunol 1985;135:207–214
32. Hirano T, Akira S, Taga T, Kishimoto T. Biological and clinical aspects of interleukin 6. Immunol Today 1990;11:443–449
33. Gahring LC, Weigle WO. The regulatory effects of cytokines on the induction of a peripheral immunologic tolerance in mice. J Immunol 1990;145:1318–1323
34. Rousset F, Garcia E, Defrance T, et al. Interleukin 10 is a potent growth and differentiation factor for activated human B lymphocytes. Proc Natl Acad Sci USA 1992;89:1890–1893
35. Konttinen YT, Hukkanen M, Kemppinen P, et al. Peptide-containing nerves in labial salivary glands in Sjögren's syndrome. Arthritis Rheum 1992;35:815–820

Oral Disease Associated with Dry Eyes

Regina H. M. Kurrasch, M.D.
Ava J. Wu, D.D.S.
Philip C. Fox, D.D.S.

A number of conditions, including amyloidosis, sarcoidosis, radiation therapy to the head, and bone marrow transplantation, may affect salivary and lacrimal tissues. However, the most common condition causing oral disease in the dry-eye patient is Sjögren's syndrome (SS), an autoimmune exocrinopathy. It should be recognized that many of the salivary gland alterations (histological and functional) seen in SS are also found in the lacrimal glands, and recent research findings concerning the pathophysiology of this disorder in one organ are likely equally applicable to the other.

SS is a systemic autoimmune disease that affects primarily the salivary and lacrimal glands, with loss of the functional glandular parenchyma resulting in decreased secretion. The most frequent presenting complaints are of dry mouth and dry eyes. There are primary and secondary forms of SS [1]. Primary SS includes the oral and ocular components without an associated connective tissue disease. Secondary SS occurs when the salivary or lacrimal gland involvement develops in the setting of a defined autoimmune connective tissue disease, most commonly rheumatoid arthritis or systemic lupus erythematosus. Although it has been described as the second most common rheumatic disease in the United States [2], the incidence of SS is unknown. Women are affected nine times more frequently than men, with the diagnosis most commonly made in middle age [1]. Diagnosis is complicated by the fact that there are currently no universally accepted objective diagnostic criteria for the exocrine components. However, some consensus has been achieved among researchers regarding minimal criteria for the diagnosis of definite SS [3]. A positive labial minor salivary gland biopsy, evidence of keratoconjunctivitis sicca (KCS) by rose bengal or fluorescein staining, and the presence of appropriate autoimmune serologies constitute the diagnosis of primary SS. Oral manifestations of SS

Selected Functions of Saliva and Potential Clinical Outcomes of Diminished Salivary Flow

Function of Saliva	Potential Outcome of Diminished Flow
Control of microbial populations	Increased caries, increased oral infections (viral, bacterial, fungal)
Lubrication of mucosa	Dysphagia, dysphonia
Maintenance of mucosal membrane integrity	Decreased protection against irritants and toxins
Buffering activity	Erosion of teeth due to pH changes, delayed dietary carbohydrate digestion
Soft-tissue repair	Impaired wound healing
Maintenance of teeth	Increased susceptibility to caries

Source: Adapted from ID Mandel, The role of saliva in maintaining oral homeostasis. J Am Dent Assoc 1989;119:298–304.

include the signs, symptoms, and complications of salivary gland dysfunction, alterations in chemosensory and motor functions of the oropharynx, and an ongoing autoimmune response, with the concomitant increased risk of development of B-cell malignancies in the glandular tissue.

■ Salivary Gland Dysfunction

Most of the oral disease seen in SS is the result of the marked salivary gland dysfunction found in many patients. Saliva plays a central role in the maintenance of oral health. Salivary gland secretions contain a wide array of protein and other factors that protect and preserve the oral hard and soft tissues [4]. Indeed, a patient with diminished salivary function is at increased risk for multiple deleterious oral sequelae (Table). Therefore, an early diagnosis so that preventive measures may be instituted is desirable.

As noted earlier, patients with SS commonly will complain of a dry mouth (xerostomia). However, xerostomia is a subjective, nonspecific complaint. It is important to recognize that not all individuals who complain of oral dryness will have salivary dysfunction and, conversely, not all individuals who have salivary dysfunction will complain of xerostomia. Multiple factors are believed to influence the sensation of oral dryness, including level of hydration, medication usage, radiation therapy involving the glands, and a host of systemic diseases [5]. Therefore, the complaint of a dry mouth, though commonly found in SS, cannot be used as a reliable diagnostic criterion for either salivary gland dysfunction or the salivary component of SS.

There are specific oral complaints found to be associated significantly with objectively measured major salivary gland hypofunction [6]. These include: (1) oral dryness while eating a meal, (2) the subjective feeling of too little saliva in the mouth, and (3) difficulty swallowing dry foods (such as a cracker) such that fluids are needed to ease swallowing [5]. Other oral complaints identified with SS include a burning sensation when eating spicy or acidic foods; food debris and lipstick sticking to the teeth; difficulty speaking for extended periods of time; oral mucosa sticking to the teeth (resulting in a "clicking" sound during speech); difficulty retaining removable dental appliances; dysphagia; decreased taste and smell; and extensive dental work [7].

Among the signs encountered in SS, bilateral, massively enlarged salivary glands have been depicted in many texts as representative of SS. Glandular enlargement is more common in patients with primary SS. Thirty to 80% of individuals will exhibit glandular enlargement over the course of their disease [8, 9]. Actually, gland enlargement is often unilateral, involves the parotid gland [10], and may not be clinically visible, but can be appreciated with bimanual palpation. The swelling may be intermittent, usually resolving without treatment over the course of 1 to 2 weeks. The possibility of bacterial infection should always be considered with the acute onset of salivary gland swelling. The gland secretion should be examined for purulence, which will be found in bacterial infection only. The occurrence of gross enlargement of salivary glands is not common and suggests the possibility of malignant transformation.

Some individuals will have a chronic enlargement of their salivary glands. Other diseases and conditions that need to be considered in the differential diagnosis are sarcoidosis, amyloidosis, granulomatous diseases, mumps, infectious mononucleosis, the acquired immunodeficiency syndrome, iodine hypersensitivity, alcoholism, and types IV and V hyperlipidemia, among others.

An increased incidence of dental decay is associated with diminished salivary function [11]. The decay often will occur despite excellent oral hygiene techniques and routine follow-up by a dentist. The caries occur in unusual locations such as the incisal edges of teeth as well as on the smooth root surfaces. In addition, SS patients exhibit marked erosion and abrasion of the teeth [12]. Prevention of caries involves the use of prescription-strength topical fluorides and frequent follow-up with a dentist.

Another frequent finding in SS is recurrent intraoral candidiasis. The presentation of intraoral candidiasis may be subtle; it can be that of classic thrush, with removable white, curdlike plaques, or an erythematous form that may be more diffuse and occurs especially beneath denture-bearing surfaces (Fig 1). Many affected patients will complain of a burning sensation when eating spicy foods. Fungal infections of the oral cavity, in the setting of inadequate salivation, may be extremely difficult to eradicate and require prolonged treatment.

Other oral signs include mucosal alterations such as partial or total papillary atrophy on the tongue, resulting in a smooth appearance, or fissuring of the tongue. In severe cases of diminished salivary flow, the

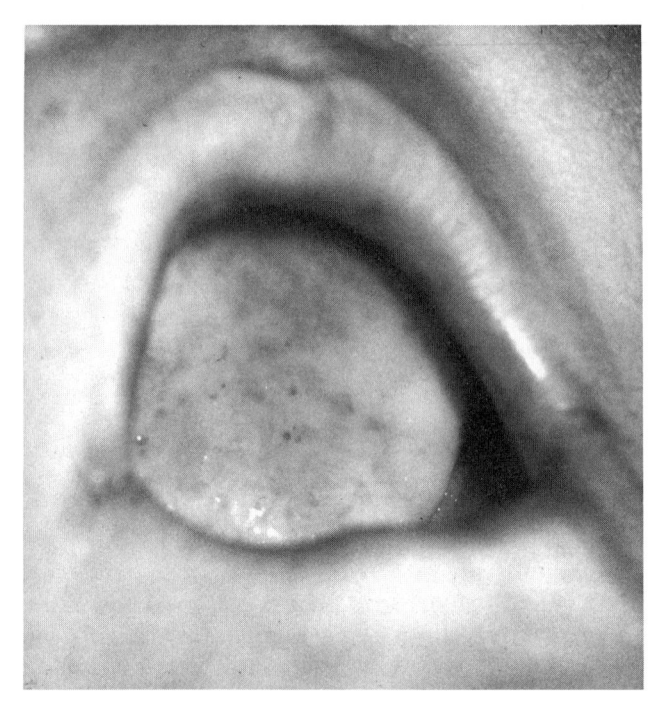

Figure 1 A patient with Sjögren's syndrome, complaining of an intraoral burning sensation, presented with mucosal erythema and angular cheilitis. Smears of the oral cavity and corners of the lips demonstrated candidal infection.

mucosa appears pale and desiccated. There may be an increased amount of intraoral debris secondary to a lack of salivary clearance.

SS patients are traditionally considered to have little to no saliva. In fact, this patient population demonstrates a wide range of salivary flow rates, from absolutely no measurable flow to seemingly normal output. The disease process affects the submandibular glands more than the parotid glands [13], and this diminished submandibular flow can be detected by the absence of salivary pooling in the floor of the mouth. Low to absent submandibular gland flow is useful for the diagnosis of SS as salivary flow rates have been inversely related to focus score and therefore serve as an indicator of disease severity [13]. Measuring salivary flow rates is valuable also for long-term monitoring of the disease process in this special population, because the noninvasive measurement of salivary flow rates is an attractive alternative to sequential lip biopsy procedures.

Changes in salivary composition (i.e., secretory proteins, electrolytes, and immunoglobulins) have been found in patients with SS [13, 14]. However, these alterations are nonspecific and can occur with other inflammatory diseases that affect the salivary glands. Compositional changes provide information regarding the functional ability of discrete areas of the salivary glands. The antimicrobial protein lactoferrin, produced by intercalated ductal and acinar cells, as well as the electrolytes Na^+ and Cl^-, secreted by acinar cells and resorbed by ductal cells, have been shown to be elevated in patients with SS [13, 14]. Although long-term monitoring of sialochemical changes could determine deterioration in gland ability as the disease progresses, to date no longitudinal studies have specifically addressed this.

■ Alterations in Oral Sensory and Motor Functions

Patients with SS exhibit alterations of chemosensory function. Although one study showed no deficit in detection of a single odor [15], another study [16] showed that almost half the patients complained of decreased smell acuity; there were defects in detection and recognition of three representative substances in almost all the patients tested. Recent studies using a 40-item forced-choice standardized recognition test have demonstrated significant impairment of olfactory identification performance in SS (J Weiffenbach, personal communication, 1993). Only 1 of 30 patients was capable of correctly identifying all 40 odors compared to 19 of 60 control subjects. Interestingly, there was no association between severity of disease and altered olfactory performance. The sensory basis for this dysfunction is not known.

SS patients often complain of a loss of taste acuity also, and this has been confirmed by demonstrated impairments of threshold taste detection and recognition and of taste intensity perception [16, 17]. Interestingly, again, taste dysfunction was not related to the salivary dysfunction found in this patient group [17].

Dysphagia is another frequent complaint in SS. It may be a result of the esophageal dysmotility found in SS, reported in up to 40% of patients [18]. In one series, 75% of the patients reported dysphagia for solids and 36% for liquids [19]. Caruso and colleagues [20] found significant differences in the duration of the oral phase of swallowing in SS patients using ultrasound imaging. Interestingly, a subset of patients with prolonged "dry" swallowing times (swallowing without additional fluid) did not show the expected decrease in swallowing duration when given a 10-ml bolus of water. The authors suggested that the chronic salivary gland hypofunction and resultant oral dryness may have altered the swallowing patterns in these patients. It is likely that the diminished salivary gland function in SS is responsible, at least in part, for the swallowing difficulties experienced by these patients.

■ Labial Salivary Gland Biopsy

Although SS is characterized clinically by disease of the major salivary glands, minor salivary glands have been shown to mirror the pathological process. Labial salivary gland biopsy has been used in the diagnosis of SS for more than 20 years and is included in all recent sets of proposed criteria because of its high diagnostic sensitivity and specificity when performed properly [21, 22]. Labial salivary gland biopsy should be considered in all patients in whom the diagnosis of SS is considered. It should be performed by those familiar with the technique and interpreted by a pathologist familiar with the histological scoring systems discussed later. Minor salivary glands exhibit significant histological changes in SS, even in the absence of major salivary gland swelling [23]. The outpatient procedure itself is simple and without serious complications, and examination of tissue allows the exclusion of other entities that can mimic SS, such as sarcoidosis, amyloidosis, and hyperlipidemias [24, 25].

Salivary gland biopsies in SS show periductal lymphocytic infiltrates and focal aggregates that replace acini while preserving the lobular architecture [23] (Fig 2). Scattered lymphocytic infiltration may be seen rarely in other pathological processes and normal aging, but acinar destruction is specific for SS [23, 26]. Myoepithelial cell hyperplasia occurs, and characteristic myoepithelial cell islands are found in major glands, although these glands are not often biopsied because of a higher operative complication rate.

Four or five minor salivary glands obtained from the inner aspect of the lower lip are embedded in the same plane for sectioning and scoring as a function of tissue area (Fig 3). Several different diagnostic scoring systems are used. The earliest system, developed by Chisholm and Mason [22], differentiates the presence of infiltrates from foci of round cells (a *focus* being defined as a collection of 50 or more cells) in the glands. Grade 4 corresponds to more than one focus per 4-mm^2 area of tissue and is diagnostic of the salivary component of SS [22], whereas the presence of a diffuse infiltrate is not.

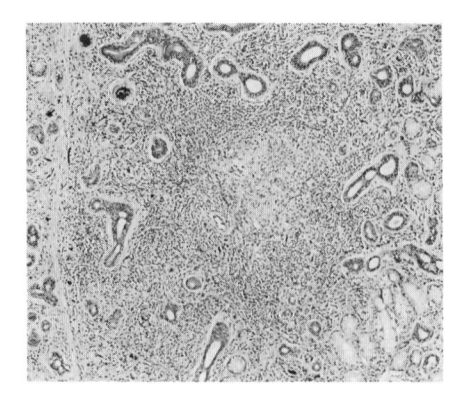

Figure 2 *The minor salivary gland from a Sjögren's syndrome patient demonstrates lymphocytic foci replacing normal glandular tissue. There is extensive loss of acinar cells and complete loss of normal architecture. (× 100)*

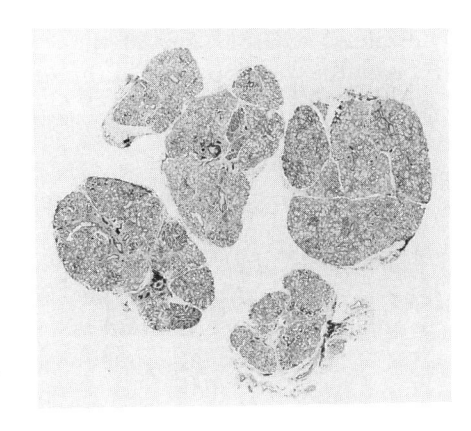

Figure 3 Minor salivary glands embedded in the same plane for diagnostic histochemical scoring. (× 10)

The Chisholm and Mason system cannot quantitate changes in focus number in patients having more than one focus, as commonly occurs in those with SS. This problem is overcome by the system of Greenspan and coworkers [26] that reports the actual number of foci per 4 mm^2 of tissue area to provide a more sensitive index of changes in inflammatory infiltrates. A focus score of greater than 1, again, is diagnostic for SS [8]. The number of foci correlates with clinical severity and tends to increase over time in SS [22, 26, 27].

The third system is the Tarpley grading system, which incorporates features from both systems, includes consideration of fibrotic changes and cell loss, and is intermediate in sensitivity [27].

■ Causes of Oral Disease

Several factors may be operative in the development of SS in the appropriate host. Genetic predisposition varies with the populations studied but has been shown to be increased in whites who are HLA-DR3+ and HLA-DQ heterozygous. Hormonal factors undoubtedly play a role, based on the marked female predominance of the disease. All factors variably contribute to the marked immune response in the salivary glandular tissue.

Viruses have been suspected to be involved in the etiology of SS. Epstein-Barr virus (EBV) infects salivary gland epithelial cells in the primary infection and remains present in a latent form. EBV DNA has been reported to be increased in SS patients with pseudolymphoma and lymphoma [28]. Human herpesvirus 6 DNA has also been detected [28]. A retroviral agent has been suspected based on the observation that a subset of Sjögren's patients has antibodies against gag proteins of human immunodeficiency virus 1 [29]. A human T-cell line cultured with SS salivary gland homogenates was observed to contain intracisternal A-type particles suggestive of the presence of a retroviral agent [30]. It is yet to be determined whether any of these viruses act as cofactors or etiological agents in the development of the malignant transformation that occurs in SS.

■ Immunological Features of the Salivary Gland

The cells infiltrating the labial salivary glands are predominantly CD4+ T lymphocytes, with lower percentages of CD8+ T cells and B cells and an absence of natural killer (NK) cells. CD4+ T cells are the first cells to appear in the inflammatory infiltrate, and their presence correlates with the extent of inflammation [23, 31, 32]. Although the mechanism of disease pathogenesis remains to be elucidated, there is strong evidence that an ongoing immune process in the salivary gland, involving infiltrating activated lymphocytes and HLA-DR+ salivary gland epithelial cells, plays a central role in autoimmunity and local tissue destruction.

The majority of T cells are alpha-, beta-antigen receptor positive [32]. They are activated by the demonstration of major histocompatibility complex class II expression but lack, or variably express, the early activation markers interleukin 2 (IL2) and transferrin receptors [33–36], and they do not appear to be actively cycling [35]. The majority of these cells are memory cells [32], that, presumably, are representative of a larger population of mucosa-associated lymphoid cells [23].

B cells account for only 10 to 25% of the infiltrate, plasma cells representing an even smaller proportion at 5 to 10% [23], but these also are activated [33]. They increase in number as the focus size increases and can form germinal centers in the major salivary glands. B cells present at the site are involved in the production of IgM and IgG, IgM and IgA rheumatoid factors, and IgA anti-SS-B antigen [37, 38]. Local synthesis of IgA rheumatoid factor contributes to the circulating pool detected in the serum of Sjögren's patients [39]. Interestingly, serum IgA rheumatoid factor titer inversely correlated with stimulated parotid flows, and concentrations of circulating IgG-IgA complexes were inversely correlated with salivary gland infiltration [40, 41], suggesting that immune complex formation either precedes or provides protection from the observed tissue destruction.

The salivary gland epithelial cells may be functioning as antigen-presenting cells within the glands as DR expression is increased, particularly around areas of lymphocytic infiltration [23, 34, 36, 42]. Upregulation of class II expression can be mediated by interferon gamma. Mitogen-stimulated T cells isolated from SS major salivary glands, but not unstimulated cells, are capable of producing interferon gamma in culture [42]. Although lymphocytes are negative, epithelial cells in areas of inflammation stain positively for interferon gamma [36, 43]. The significance of this is not known. Infiltrating lymphocytes and epithelial cells are variably positive for interferon alpha and beta but lack either IL2 or IL2 receptor [36]. Therefore, at the present time, no characteristic pattern of cytokine expression in the lesions of SS patients has been demonstrated. The exact pathogenic mechanism of this local immune response, as well as its contribution to local tissue destruction, remains to be determined.

■ Malignant Transformation

SS is unique among the autoimmune diseases in that patients have been noted to have a 44-fold increased risk for the development of non-Hodgkin's lymphoma and other B-cell malignancies [44]. The salivary glands are the most common site for these malignancies, and chronic salivary gland swelling, lymphadenopathy, and splenomegaly are high risk factors. This has led to the hypothesis that SS is part of a spectrum of diseases of lymphoproliferation. Indeed, it has been noted that a significant percentage of SS patients without obvious malignant disease have chronic B-cell clonal proliferations as detected by serum and urine paraproteins [45]. As the salivary glandular infiltrates increase in size, and T cells remain predominant, the lesion is defined as a *pseudolymphoma*. When T cells are replaced by a monotypical B-cell infiltrate, the lesion progresses from pre-lymphoma to frank non-Hodgkin's lymphoma. Salivary gland lymphomas are typical of those that develop in other mucosa-associated lymphoid tissues, such as the stomach [46, 47]; they have an indolent course and may even remit spontaneously. Based on these studies and our experience, it is our recommendation that all patients with persistent salivary gland enlargement undergo salivary gland biopsy, with appropriate immunohistochemical staining for early diagnosis and treatment of B-cell malignancies.

The progression of B-cell infiltration into lesions of the salivary glands has been well-studied. Serial biopsies have documented that B cells bearing a cross-reactive idiotype shared by rheumatoid factor paraproteins in Waldenstrom's macroglobulinemia were initially present and increased in number until overt lymphoma developed [48]. Some of these B cells bear the bcl-2 t(14;18) translocation found in non-Hodgkin's lymphomas at other sites [49]. Surprisingly, benign lesions, with polyclonal B-cell infiltrates by immunohistochemistry, have been shown to have detectable immunoglobulin rearrangements, indicating that even in early lesions, a clonal expansion of 1 to 3% of B cells can occur. Furthermore, different B-cell clones can expand at different times in the course of the disease, possibly as a result of abnormal immune surveillance [50, 51].

■ Treatment of Oral Disease

The treatment of SS is symptomatic. Salivary substitutes are available, but we find that they are not well-accepted by patients. Their preference seems to be water, and many patients will carry a small bottle from which they can sip throughout the day. In addition, sugarless hard candies and gum may be used to stimulate salivary flow.

Clinical trials of various salivary stimulants have been completed. Pilocarpine, a secretory stimulant, has been found to ameliorate the feeling of oral dryness and increase salivary flow rate in SS patients who have remaining functional parenchyma [52]. Bromhexine and anethole-trithione are two additional stimulants that have been tested in Europe and Canada, but their efficacy has not yet been proved. Additional pharmaceuticals that have been used or tested or are currently in clinical trials include antirheumatics, steroids, and cytotoxic agents [53, 54].

The ideal medication for the treatment of candidiasis in this population is the use of powdered nystatin, containing no fermentable sugars or carbohydrates, that may be reconstituted in water and sprinkled directly into the oral cavity or onto a denture. Other antifungal preparations contain substantial concentrations of sugars that can promote tooth decay in this susceptible population. Finally, as noted earlier, patients require increased dental surveillance and should be placed on supplemental fluorides.

■ References

1. Bloch KJ, Buchanan WW, Wohl MJ, et al. Sjögren's syndrome: a clinical pathological and serological study of sixty-two cases. Medicine 1965;44:187–231
2. Lane CH, Fauci AS. Sjögren's syndrome. In: Wilson JD, Brunwald E, Petersdorf RG, et al., eds. Harrison's principles of internal medicine, ed 12, vol 2. New York: McGraw-Hill, 1990
3. Fox RI, Robinson CA, Curd JG, et al. Sjögren's syndrome: proposed criteria for classification. Arthritis Rheum 1986;29:577–585
4. Mandel ID. The role of saliva in maintaining oral homeostasis. J Am Dent Assoc 1989;119:298–304
5. Fox PC, van der Ven PF, Sonies BC, et al. Xerostomia: evaluation of a symptom with increasing significance. J Am Dent Assoc 1985;110:518–525
6. Fox PC, Busch KA, Baum BJ. Subjective reports of xerostomia and objective measures of salivary gland performance. J Am Dent Assoc 1987;115:581–584
7. Daniels TE, Fox PC. Salivary and oral components of Sjögren's syndrome. Rheum Dis Clin North Am 1992;18:571–589
8. Daniels TE. Labial salivary gland biopsy in Sjögren's syndrome: assessment as a diagnostic criterion in 362 suspected cases. Arthritis Rheum 1984;27:147–156
9. Moutsopoulos HM, Webber BL, Vlagopoulos TP, et al. Difference in the clinical manifestations of sicca syndrome in the presence and absence of rheumatoid arthritis. Am J Med 1979;66:733–736
10. Whaley K, Webb J, McAvoy BA, et al. Sjögren's syndrome: 2 clinical associations and clinical phenomena. Q J Med 1973;42:513–548
11. Pappas AS, Joshi A, MacDonald SL, et al. Caries prevalence in xerostomic individuals. J Can Dent Assoc 1993;59:171–179
12. Atkinson JC, Fox PC. Sjögren's syndrome: oral and dental considerations. J Am Dent Assoc 1993;124:74–86
13. Atkinson JC, Travis WD, Pillemer SR, et al. Major salivary gland function in pri-

mary Sjögren's syndrome and its relationship to clinical features. J Rheumatol 1990; 17:318–322
14. Stuchell RN, Mandel ID, Baurmash H. Clinical utilization of sialochemistry in Sjögren's syndrome. J Oral Pathol 1984;13:303–309
15. Rasmussen N, Brofeldt S, Manthorpe R. Smell and nasal findings in patients with primary Sjögren's syndrome. Scand J Rheumatol 1986;61:142–145
16. Henkin RI, Talal N, Larson AL, Mattern CFT. Abnormalities of taste and smell in Sjögren's syndrome. Ann Intern Med 1972;76:375–383
17. Weiffenbach JM, Atkinson JC, Fox PC, Baum BJ. Taste deficits of Sjögren's syndrome [abstr]. J Dent Res 1987;66:202
18. Tsianos EB, Vasakos S, Drosos AA, et al. The gastrointestinal involvement in primary Sjögren's syndrome. Scand J Rheumatol Suppl 1986;61:151–155
19. Kjellen G, Fransson SG, Lindstrom F, et al. Esophageal function, radiography, and dysphagia in Sjögren's syndrome. Dig Dis Sci 1986;31:225–229
20. Caruso AJ, Sonies BC, Atkinson JC, Fox PC. Objective measures of swallowing in patients with primary Sjögren's syndrome. Dysphagia 1989;4:101–105
21. Daniels TE. Salivary histopathology in diagnosis of Sjögren's syndrome. Scand J Rheumatol Suppl 1986;61:36–43
22. Chisholm DM, Mason DK. Labial salivary gland biopsy in Sjögren's syndrome. J Clin Pathol 1968;21:656–660
23. Fox RI, Howell FV, Bone RC, Michelson P. Primary Sjögren's syndrome: clinical and immunopathologic features. Semin Arthritis Rheum 1984;14:77–105
24. Skopouli FN, Drosos AA, Papaioannou T, Moutsopoulos HM. Preliminary diagnostic criteria for Sjögren's syndrome. Scand J Rheumatol Suppl 1986;61:22–25
25. Speight PM, Cruchley A, Williams DM. Epithelial HLA-DR expression in labial salivary glands in Sjögren's syndrome and non-specific sialadenitis. J Oral Pathol Med 1989;18:178–183
26. Greenspan JS, Daniels TE, Talal N, Sylvester RA. The histopathology of Sjögren's syndrome in labial salivary gland biopsies. Oral Surg Oral Med Oral Pathol 1974;37:217–229
27. Tarpley TM, Anderson LG, White CL. Minor salivary gland involvement in Sjögren's syndrome. Oral Surg Oral Med Oral Pathol 1974;37:64–73
28. Fox RI, Saito I, Chan EK, et al. Viral genomes in lymphomas of patients with Sjögren's syndrome. J Autoimmun 1989;2:449–455
29. Talal N, Garry R, Alexander SS, et al. Detection of serum antibodies to retroviral proteins in patients with primary Sjögren's syndrome (autoimmune exocrinopathy). Arthritis Rheum 1990;33:1866–1871
30. Garry RF, Fermin CD, Hart DJ. Detection of a human intracisternal A-type retroviral particle antigenically related to HIV. Science 1990;341:72–74
31. Fox RI, Hugli TE, Lanier LL, et al. Salivary gland lymphocytes in primary Sjögren's syndrome lack lymphocyte subsets defined by Leu-7 and Leu-11 antigens. J Immunol 1985;135:207–214
32. Skoupouli FN, Fox PC, Galanpoulou V, et al. T cell subpopulations in the labial minor salivary gland histopathologic lesion of Sjögren's syndrome. J Rheumatol 1991;18:210–214
33. Fox RI, Adamson TC, Fong S, Robinson CA. Lymphocyte phenotype and function in pseudolymphoma associated with Sjögren's syndrome. J Clin Invest 1983;72:52–62
34. Jonsson R, Klarekog L, Backman K, Tarkowski A. Expression of HLA-D-locus (DP, DQ, DR)–coded antigens, beta-2-microglobulin, and the interleukin 2 receptor in Sjögren's syndrome. Clin Immunol Immunopathol 1987;45:235–243
35. Segerberg-Konttinen M, Bergroth V, Jungell P, et al. T lymphocyte activation state in the minor salivary glands of patients with Sjögren's syndrome. Ann Rheum Dis 1987;46:649–653

36. Rowe D, Griffiths M, Stewart J, et al. HLA class I and II, interferon, interleukin 2, and the interleukin 2 receptor expression on labial biopsy specimens from patients with Sjögren's syndrome. Ann Rheum Dis 1987;46:580–586
37. Talal N, Asofsky R, Lightbody P. Immunoglobulin synthesis by salivary gland lymphoid cells in Sjögren's syndrome. J Clin Invest 1970;49:49–54
38. Anderson LG, Cummings NA, Asofsky R, et al. Salivary gland immunoglobulin and rheumatoid factor synthesis in Sjögren's syndrome. Am J Med 1972;53:456–463
39. Elkon KB, Delacroix DL, Gharvari AE, et al. Immunoglobulin A and polymeric IgA rheumatoid factors in systemic sicca syndrome: partial characterization. J Immunol 1982;129:576–581
40. Atkinson JC, Fox PC, Travis WD, et al. IgA rheumatoid factor and IgA containing immune complexes in primary Sjögren's syndrome. J Rheumatol 1989;16:1205–1210
41. Atkinson JC, Travis WD, Slocum L, et al. Serum anti-SS-B/La and IgA rheumatoid factor are markers of salivary gland disease activity in primary Sjögren's syndrome. Arthritis Rheum 1992;35:1368–1372
42. Fox RI, Bumol T, Fantozzi R, et al. Expression of histocompatibility antigen HLA-DR by salivary gland epithelial cells in Sjögren's syndrome. Arthritis Rheum 1986;29:1105–1111
43. Hedfors E, Lindahl G. Variation of MHC Class I and II antigen expression in relation to lymphocytic infiltrates and interferon-gamma positive cells. J Rheumatol 1990;17:743–750
44. Kassan SS, Thomas TL, Moutsopoulos HM, et al. Increased risk of lymphoma in sicca syndrome. Ann Intern Med 1978;89:888–892
45. Moutsopoulos HM, Costello R, Drosos AA, et al. Demonstration and identification of monoclonal proteins in the urine of patients with Sjögren's syndrome. Ann Rheum Dis 1985;44:109–112
46. Schmid U, Lennert K, Gloor F. Immunosialadenitis (Sjögren's syndrome) and lymphoproliferation. Clin Exp Rheumatol 1989;7:175–180
47. Diss TC, Peng H, Wotherspoon AC, et al. Brief report: a single neoplastic clone in sequential biopsy specimens from a patient with primary gastric-mucosa-associated lymphoid tissue lymphoma and Sjögren's syndrome. N Engl J Med 1993;329:172–175
48. Fox RI, Carson DA, Chen P, Fong S. Characterization of a cross-reactive idiotype in Sjögren's syndrome. Scand J Rheumatol Suppl 1986;61:83–88
49. Pisa EK, Pisa P, Kang H, Fox RI. High frequency of the t(14;18) translocation in salivary gland lymphomas from Sjögren's syndrome patients. J Exp Med 1991;174:1245–1250
50. Fishleder A, Tubbs R, Hesse B, Levine H. Uniform detection of immunoglobulin-gene rearrangement in benign lymphoepithelial lesions. N Engl J Med 1987;316:1118–1121
51. Freimark B, Fantozzi R, Bone R, et al. Detection of clonally expanded salivary gland lymphocytes in Sjögren's syndrome. Arthritis Rheum 1989;32:859–869
52. Fox PC, Atkinson JC, Macynski AA, et al. Pilocarpine treatment of salivary gland hypofunction and dry mouth (xerostomia). Arch Intern Med 1991;151:1149–1152
53. Fox PC, Datiles M, Atkinson JC, et al. Prednisone and piroxicam for treatment of primary Sjögren's syndrome. Clin Exp Rheumatol 1993;11:149–156
54. Fox RI, Chan E, Benton L, et al. Treatment of primary Sjögren's syndrome with hydroxychloroquine. Am J Med 1988;85(suppl 4A):62–67

Management of the Dry-Eye Patient

Michael A. Lemp, M.D.

Treatment of the dry eye involves the challenges and frustrations associated with the management of a chronic disease. Frustration on the part of both the practitioner and the patient can be minimized if the goals of the treatment are clearly understood at the outset. In this case, the goals are the preservation of vision and the relief of discomfort. It should be emphasized to patients that there is generally no cure for their affliction but, with proper attention and an adequate treatment regimen, it is likely that good vision can be preserved throughout life and a considerable degree of comfort afforded. Successful management of a chronic condition such as dry eyes involves a partnership between physician and patient in which trust, conscientious application of therapeutic measures, and careful experimentation are all important ingredients.

■ Definition of the Dry Eye

The term *dry eyes* is used somewhat generically to describe a variety of ocular disorders of diverse pathogenesis that share as a common manifestation signs and symptoms of ocular surface disease [1]. The manifestations of ocular surface disease arise from decreased aqueous tear secretion, abnormalities of conjunctival mucin secretion, meibomian gland dysfunction, eyelid surface abnormalities (e.g., seventh nerve paresis, symblephara of the conjunctiva, and other eyelid abnormalities such as exposure keratitis), primary ocular surface disease itself (e.g., decreased sensation of the cornea), and other conditions that place stress on the tear film such as the wearing of contact lenses and primary inflammatory disease of the ocular surface (e.g., Sjögren's syndrome).

Aqueous tear secretion decreases with aging. This is not a major problem for most individuals but, in some patients, tear production decreases sufficiently to give rise to irritative symptoms. The relative roles of decreased tear production by the lacrimal glands and increased evaporation of tear film is, as yet, controversial. Paralleling the decrease in tear secretion in the lacrimal glands, however, is a decrease in certain enzymatic constituents of tears—lysozyme, lactoferrin, and beta-lysin. These enzymes provide protection against infection and thus, in keratoconjunctivitis sicca (KCS), there is a decreased resistance of the external eye to infection. Recent studies have implicated both estrogen and androgen effects on tear production [2]. Additionally, experimental evidence with the use of antiestrogen drugs such as tamoxifen [3] and surgical oophorectomy in rats [4] has shown that both of these lead to atrophic changes in the lacrimal glands and in the glycoprotein content of ocular mucin. Additional evidence of the hormonal regulation of tear production and ocular surface changes is the observation that the human conjunctiva responds to the menstrual cycle with changes in ocular surface cell morphology [5].

Most cases of KCS occur in the absence of any identifiable systemic disease. There is, however, an association between systemic inflammatory disease and KCS in patients with Sjögren's syndrome. In patients with bona fide Sjögren's disease there is, in addition to decreased aqueous tearing, a primary inflammatory process on the ocular surface, and a subset of these patients can have severe ocular inflammatory problems such as scleritis, episcleritis, rheumatoid nodules, and corneal ulceration.

Recent work has identified small molecular components of the tear film, such as growth factors and retinol. It has been suggested that these components are synthesized by the lacrimal glands at a low level and act on the ocular surface to help regulate normal turnover of corneal and conjunctival epithelial cells. A breakdown in the synthesis of one or more of these components may play a role in the pathogenesis of ocular surface disease in some dry-eye states [6].

Abnormalities in the secretion of the meibomian glands of the eyelids are associated with changes in the ocular surface. Meibomian gland dysfunction—which is characterized by inspissation of the glands and a change from clear to turbid secretion, thick columnar secretions, or complete obstruction of the meibomian gland openings—have been associated with increased evaporation from the ocular surface [7]. The leads to the development of a so-called pseudo–dry eye, manifested by increased tonicity in the tear film and ocular surface disease.

Clearly, a variety of conditions affecting the external eye can result in changes in the tear film and ocular surface abnormalities, all of which fall under the rubric the dry eye.

■ Therapeutic Options

Artificial Tear Preparations

The mainstay of therapy for dry eyes is the replacement of deficient tear production with tear substitutes [8]. These substitutes have a long history. It was discovered initially that the use of nonisotonic solutions was associated with discomfort. Therefore, normal saline was used and was found to provide immediate relief in many cases. This relief, however, was short-lived. Additives were developed and used initially to thicken the tear substitutes, which was believed to prolong their action. Early examples of this type of artificial tear include those containing cellulose ethers such as methylcellulose and hydroxymethylcellulose. These thick preparations did indeed last somewhat longer than normal saline, but they tended to blur vision. Thus, they proved to be of real but limited value. Further developments in the 1960s included the use of polyvinyl alcohol, a film-forming polymer that was believed to have an attraction to the ocular surface. It was not until the early 1970s that a scientific basis for the development of polymer-containing artificial tears was accomplished. A number of products containing polymers with adsorptive properties for the ocular surface were developed, including Tears Naturale and Hypotears, both of which were formulated in a relatively nonviscous form. These demonstrated evidence of their effects in the eye for up to 1½ hours after instillation.

A wide variety of artificial tear preparations now exist, among which are preparations containing adsorptive polymers, some viscous and others nonviscous. In general, patients tolerate nonviscous products better. One product, Hypotears, is formulated in a hypotonic concentration. It is believed that this counteracts the hypertonicity of the tear film in KCS and therefore aids in rehydrating the ocular surface. It has not, however, been demonstrated that this rehydration of the ocular surface actually is facilitated by the use of hypotonic solutions.

A newer type of artificial tear preparation (Bion Tear) employs a unique electrolyte-based formulation that has been shown to be beneficial to the ocular surface in animal studies. Another new product, Aqua Site, employs a viscous droplet that is instilled into the inferior cul-de-sac and is reported to act as a reservoir replenishing the preocular tear film for a sustained period. Alternatively, a tear gel has been used in Europe for some time, and a similar product (Tear Gel) is under active investigation in the United States. Other attempts to devise a beneficial artificial tear include the use of sodium hyaluronate (Healon) solution, which is made by diluting the viscous preparation used in intraocular surgery. The stability of these diluted products is still under investigation, though some practitioners already recommend them highly.

Approximately 15 years ago, sustained-release artificial tear inserts (Lacriserts) became available (Fig 1). These 5-mg hydroxypropylcellulose rods dissolve on contact with the ocular surface and release a viscous watery coating. The effects of one of these inserts can last 6 to 12 hours after insertion. The inserts provide a thick precorneal tear film and are particularly useful in KCS with an exposure component [9, 10]. Drawbacks include the development of a shimmering vision, particularly 2 to 3 hours after instillation, which is noted most on attempted reading. The probable

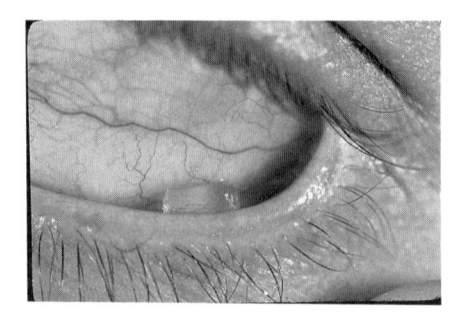

Figure 1 Undissolved Lacrisert. *(Reprinted with permission from Lemp [19].)*

cause is the very thick tear film noted just over the inferior eyelid margin. Lacriserts are also expensive and require some manual dexterity on the part of the patient to accomplish their safe insertion. They require some degree of hydration to work and, in patients with severe tear deficiencies, Lacriserts must be used in conjunction with other artificial tear preparations to initiate the dissolving process. Their cost and the difficulty in managing them has limited their usefulness. Lacriserts are most effective in patients with moderate to severe symptoms who cannot be adequately managed with frequent instillation of artificial tears.

The Role of Preservatives in Corneal Disease and KCS The preparation of artificial tear solutions is complicated. To ensure a long shelf life and stability of these preparations, manufacturers commonly employ, in addition to polymers, a variety of stabilizers and preservatives. Preservatives retard the growth of microbial organisms while also usually having toxic effects on all cells including those of the ocular surface. The concentration of preservatives used in artificial tear solutions is generally sufficiently low that the toxic effects on the cornea and conjunctival epithelium are minimal. In an already compromised epithelium, however, such as occurs often in KCS, the frequent use of drops containing preservatives can induce a significant degree of iatrogenic surface disease. The most commonly employed preservatives are benzalkonium chloride, chlorobutanol, thimerosal, and chlorhexidine, the most toxic of which is benzalkonium chloride. This cationic detergent emulsifies lipids of cell walls. Chronic use of preservative-containing solutions, particularly in an otherwise compromised ocular surface, can result in irritation, lacrimation, hyperemia, photophobia, and even corneal edema. Clinically, the following conditions have been associated with the use of benzalkonium chloride–containing drops: punctate keratitis, gray corneal epithelial haze, pseudomembrane formation in the conjunctiva, a decrease in corneal epithelial microvilli and, possibly, a delay in corneal wound healing.

Over the past several years, a number of preservative-free products have been formulated. These products employ unit-dose dispensing; the small dispensing vials are used once and then discarded. Although this adds to the cost of the product, in patients using artificial tears more frequently than three to four times daily, it probably is wiser to recommend the use of preservative-free artificial tears to avoid the likelihood of worsening the ocular surface condition from preservative toxicity.

Lubricants

The relative roles of hydration and lubrication in the pathogenesis of ocular surface disease associated with KCS are still undetermined. It is known, however, that many patients with KCS develop problems during the night and on awakening, presumably owing to the further decrease of tear production during sleep. The application of an ointment before retiring (e.g., Lacrilube or Dualube) provides a long-lasting means of increasing lubricity between the eyelid and the ocular surface during sleep. Approximately 1/8 inch of ointment is sufficient to provide lubrication during the night without substantially blurring vision the following morning. The use of lubricating agents is an adjunct to the use of artificial tears throughout the day.

Tear Stimulation

Laboratory investigation over the past 5 years has elucidated many of the mechanisms operative in tear secretion in the lacrimal glands. As a result of these studies, a number of small molecular naturally occurring chemicals have been identified that stimulate lacrimal gland secretion. These agents, and some analogs, have been investigated in laboratory animals and in human studies. While they appear promising, as yet no tear preparation containing one of these lacrimomimetic agents has been approved for use in the United States. Bromhexine has been widely used abroad, both topically and systemically.

Tear Preservation

It is possible to take measures to preserve existing scanty tear production. The most commonly used approach involves occlusion of the puncta leading into the canaliculi and nasolacrimal sac and duct. The decision to occlude all the puncta should not be taken lightly. In many patients, particularly those who are young, KCS tends to have a waxing and waning course. A hasty decision to occlude all the puncta permanently can lead to the development of epiphora, which can be very disturbing to the patient.

Nonetheless, there has been a resurgence of interest in this procedure over the last several years as a useful way of managing patients with more severe forms of KCS. A silicone plug (Freeman plug) has been developed that can be inserted into the inferior and superior puncta after punctal dilatation (Fig 2). This can be used as a temporary measure or as a means

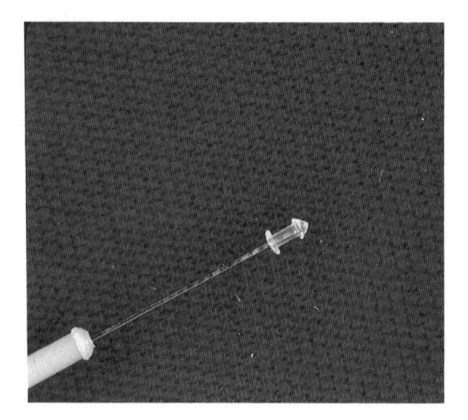

Figure 2 *Freeman punctal plug. (Reprinted with permission from Lemp [19].)*

of assessing the effectiveness of punctal occlusions. New designs of these plugs have recently been introduced to accommodate different-sized puncta. More recently, intracanalicular collagen rods have been developed. These temporary occlusive devices can be inserted within the canaliculi and will dissolve within approximately two to three days, thus allowing a trial period in which the advisability of more permanent punctal occlusion can be assessed.

Permanent punctal occlusion usually involves the application of heat to the puncta to effect a permanent seal. This has traditionally been done with the use of a cautery. A substantial degree of heat must be applied throughout the extensive portion of the superior part of the canaliculus; sufficient epithelium must be destroyed so that a good scar will result. Light application of cautery to the openings of the puncta usually results in only temporary occlusion; these areas generally open within 1 week's time. Application to the puncta of a fine wire tip of a cautery instrument such as a Hyfrecator (Birtcher Corporation, Los Angeles, CA) with strong current after use of local anesthetic is recommended for permanent closure. More recently, some have advocated the use of argon lasers to produce the same effect, but no advantage in the use of this expensive new technology has been demonstrated. Indeed, the recent literature has demonstrated that the use of lasers is associated with a higher rate of reopening of the puncta [11]. The decision to occlude the puncta permanently should be made only when there is evidence of persistent moderate to severe decrease in tear production with evidence of significant ocular surface disease. Occlusion of the inferior puncta only is associated with much less risk of the production of epiphora. The subject of punctal occlusion is addressed fully in the chapter by Dr Lamberts in this issue.

Studies have suggested that increased evaporation is one mechanism that produces ocular surface disease associated with dry eyes [12]. In more severe cases, the use of tightly fitting swimming goggles or other types of tightly fitting eyewear may decrease evaporation around the eye and may, therefore, be useful. This treatment modality should be limited to severe cases.

Antiinflammatory Therapy

Low-grade inflammation, including chronic lymphocytic infiltration, has been demonstrated in specimens of the lacrimal glands from patients with KCS. This inflammation is long-standing and low-grade and so, in general, antiinflammatory treatment has no place in the management of these patients with KCS. In the subset of patients with KCS who have Sjögren's disease and, therefore, primary inflammation of the ocular surface, immunomodulating agents may well be useful. This is particularly true in those patients who show moderate to severe inflammation and other signs of ocular surface involvement such as rheumatoid nodules, scleritis, and corneal ulcers. The use of topical immunomodulating agents such as cyclosporine may be appropriate for managing these severe problems.

Other conditions, such as erythema multiforme and ocular pemphigoid, that cause drying of the ocular surface may also warrant antiinflammatory treatment. Severe cases, particularly of ocular pemphigoid, have been shown to respond well to systemic treatment with antimetabolites [13]. Because of the side effects of antimetabolites, such therapy should be confined to those patients with severe, extensive ocular surface disease and should always be undertaken under the guidance of an internist skilled and experienced in the use of these agents.

Preservation of a Moist Surface

Occasionally useful in managing dry-eye conditions is the attempt to reverse some of the desiccation seen on the corneal surface, which can be accomplished with bandage soft contact lenses. These water-filled lenses provide a moist covering and exchange some of their fluid with the epithelium, thus playing a role in rehydrating desiccated epithelium. Bandage contact lenses are particularly useful in cases of filamentary keratitis as they have been associated with the rapid dissolution of the filaments and prompt relief of severe discomfort.

The use of bandage hydrophilic lenses does, however, carry with it several risks. These lenses must be used in conjunction with artificial tear preparations as they tend to dry out quickly. A desiccated bandage contact lens in a dry eye constitutes an irritable foreign body that can worsen the situation (Fig 3). Virtually all the artificial tear preparations have been shown to be compatible with instillation into the eye containing a bandage contact lens. The preservatives contained in these preparations do not seem to penetrate the bandage lens in any appreciable amount in vivo.

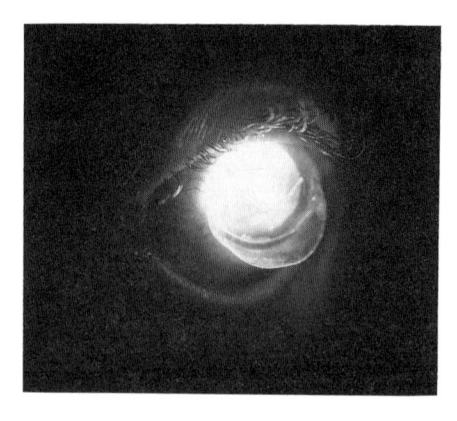

Figure 3 Desiccated bandage contact lens in patient with keratoconjunctivitis sicca and exposure keratitis. (Reprinted with permission from Lemp [19].)

The situation with preservative-containing solutions outside the eye is very different. Preservatives are drawn out rapidly by the lens from a lens soaked in preservative-containing solutions, which can cause severe chemical keratitis. Consequently, preservative-free artificial tear preparations in conjunction with a bandage contact lens is the recommended form of treatment.

Bandage contact lenses are associated with a high rate of complications in patients with KCS. Deposits occur frequently with use of these lenses in KCS, being almost a constant problem in many patients (Fig 4). The most serious complication associated with the use of bandage lenses in dry eyes is the development of infection. Because the dry eye has severely compromised ocular surface defense mechanisms, placing a moist covering over the cornea with sequestered tear film beneath it provides a setting in which bacterial infections can flourish. It has been demonstrated that bacteria attach to hydrophilic contact lenses [14] and the use of prophylactic antibiotic drops does not guarantee the control of infection but may, in fact, encourage the emergence of antibiotic-resistant organisms. Finally, the development of a serious corneal ulcer with endophthalmitis is a very real danger associated with hydrophilic lens use in dry eyes (Fig 5).

The considerable risks associated with bandage soft contact lens wear

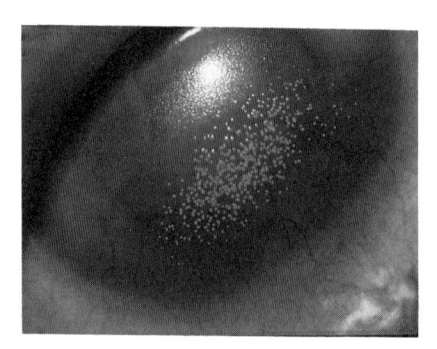

Figure 4 Deposits on bandage contact lens in patient with keratoconjunctivitis sicca. (Reprinted with permission from Lemp [19].)

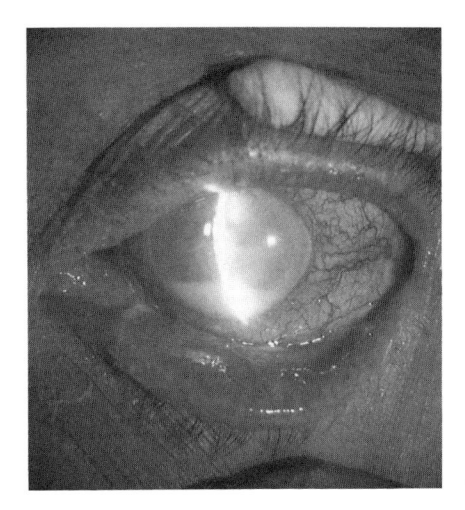

Figure 5 *Endophthalmitis associated with bandage contact lens wear in patient with keratoconjunctivitis sicca. (Reprinted with permission from Lemp [19].)*

in dry eyes leads me to recommend their use in only a very small number of patients with intractable filamentary keratitis that cannot be managed by any other treatment modality and in only those patients who are observant and vigilant in hygiene and understand the risks involved.

Surface Treatment

The use of artificial tears, lubricants, bandage lenses, and antiinflammatory therapy are all directed to the improvement of the ocular surface. Topical application of retinoids has been advocated and reported to be useful in reversing cellular changes noted in the conjunctiva of patients with some forms of dry eyes [15]. No randomized, well-designed clinical trial, however, has demonstrated a statistically significant benefit in the use of retinoid-containing topical preparations. This remains under investigation.

Decreasing Tear Viscosity

Some patients with KCS have particularly viscous, stringy mucus that may be associated with filaments or coarse mucous plaques on the ocular surface, which appear to be major sources of irritation and discomfort. The use of a 10 to 20% solution of acetylcysteine four to five times daily can help decrease the viscosity of mucus on the ocular surface. The solution itself tends to be irritating on application; a milder 10% solution is more tolerable in this regard. Acetylcysteine is fairly expensive and prepared without a preservative, thereby limiting its shelf life. In practice, however, bottles made up and stored in the refrigerator may be safely used over a period of 3 to 4 weeks. This, in addition to artificial tears and any other treatment, can help improve the symptomatology in patients in whom particularly viscous, stringy mucus is noted in the tear film.

Estrogens

The prevalence of KCS in menopausal and postmenopausal women has raised the question of possible association with estrogen deficiency. As noted earlier, recent evidence has strengthened the link between hormonal dysfunction and ocular surface disease. Systemically administered estrogens have been used for decades by clinicians in the management of some cases of dry eyes. Anecdotal reports of efficacy have appeared. Recently, early beneficial results of a topical estrogen-containing preparation have been reported, but further research is required before the role of this type of therapy can be established [16].

Surgery

In an attempt to deal with some of the more severe types of dry-eye syndromes, a number of different surgical modalities have been employed. Among these is mucous membrane grafting from buccal mucosa, which is particularly useful in patients with severely scarred conjunctiva such as occurs after chemical burns, ocular pemphigoid, and the Stevens-Johnson syndrome. The failure rate is very high, however. More successful is autotransplantation of areas of normal conjunctiva from one eye to another, particularly in cases of chemical burns. Another surgical procedure that has been employed is parotid duct transplantation, in which ducts leading from the parotid gland are transplanted so that they empty out to the conjunctival surface [17]. The parotid secretion is different from that of normal tear secretion and is much more copious. Complications associated with the copious secretion of such a foreign fluid into the ocular surface include a strange type of epiphora, which has led to the virtual abandonment of this procedure.

In severe types of cicatricial disease such as ocular pemphigoid and the Stevens-Johnson syndrome, severe trachoma, and chemical burns in which scarring has been extensive, corneal prostheses have been implanted. Some of these have resulted in spectacular improvements in vision, but practically all these corneal implants have ultimately been extruded, and loss of the eye is not infrequent [18].

The use of a lateral blepharoplasty (tarsorrhaphy) has enjoyed a resurgence of interest in recent years [19]. In patients with severe ocular surface disease, particularly persistent epithelial defects and noninfectious corneal ulcers, a tarsorrhaphy can be extremely useful. One theory supporting its use in patients with KCS attributes efficacy to decreasing the exposed surface of the eye. Because evaporation has been implicated as a causative mechanism in the desiccation of the ocular surface, decreasing the area available for evaporation seems a reasonable and innocuous procedure.

■ Choosing the Proper Method of Treatment

It can be seen that a number of measures are available for managing various manifestations of dry eyes. One of the most frequently asked questions is which type of treatment modality is most appropriate for a given patient. I have developed a scheme to aid the practitioner in making this decision. Figure 6 is a modified Latin square in which the coordinates plot the results of change for a number of clinical tests used in the diagnosis of dry eyes. This is, at best, a semiquantitative notation designed to aid the practitioner in assessing the severity of disease. When values are plotted and the intersecting coordinates are identified, one generally can divide patients into three broad categories graded 1 through 3. Patients showing rose bengal staining of 0 to 1 and a Schirmer test result of 4 mm of wetting without anesthetic over 5 minutes would clearly fall into the grade 1 category. In contrast, a patient with 3+ rose bengal staining and up to 1 mm of wetting on the Schirmer test without anesthetic falls into grade 3. Alternatively, tear film osmolarity or tear film breakup time (a measure of tear film instability) can be used. Figure 7 suggests some appropriate treatment regimens for each stage in the disease process. All these are merely general guidelines, but they do suggest what will work for most patients.

■ Comments

With interest and attention on the part of the physician and conscientious compliance by the patient, the vast majority of patients with dry eyes

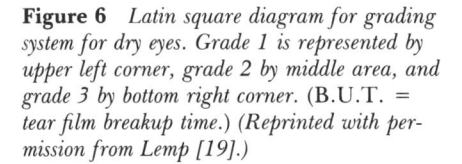

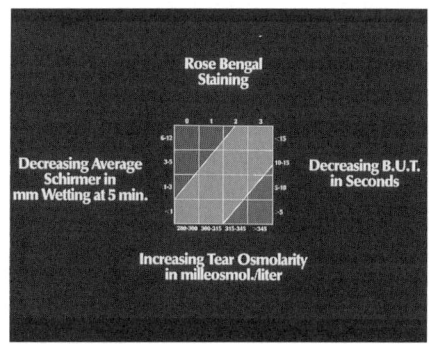

Figure 6 *Latin square diagram for grading system for dry eyes. Grade 1 is represented by upper left corner, grade 2 by middle area, and grade 3 by bottom right corner. (B.U.T. = tear film breakup time.) (Reprinted with permission from Lemp [19].)*

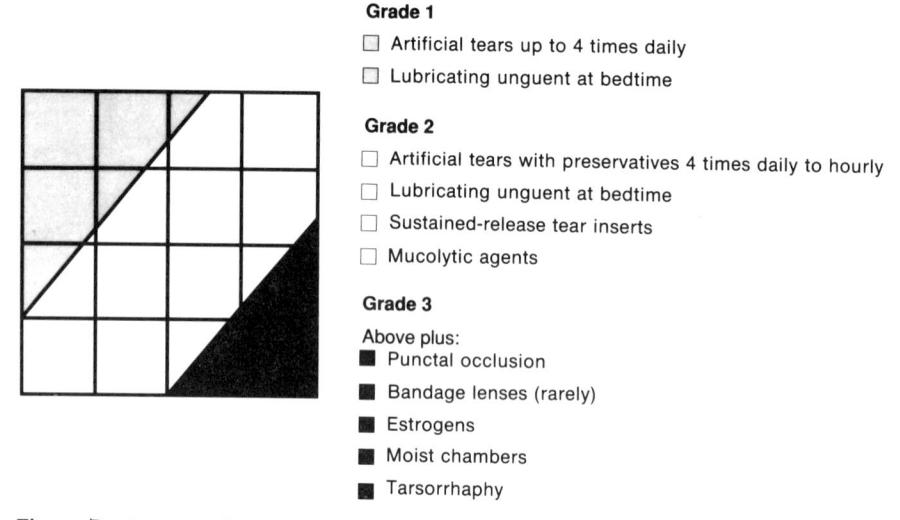

Figure 7 *Recommended treatment modalities for dry eyes. (Reprinted with permission from Lemp [19].)*

Grade 1
- ☐ Artificial tears up to 4 times daily
- ☐ Lubricating unguent at bedtime

Grade 2
- ☐ Artificial tears with preservatives 4 times daily to hourly
- ☐ Lubricating unguent at bedtime
- ☐ Sustained-release tear inserts
- ☐ Mucolytic agents

Grade 3
Above plus:
- ■ Punctal occlusion
- ■ Bandage lenses (rarely)
- ■ Estrogens
- ■ Moist chambers
- ■ Tarsorrhaphy

can be successfully managed, maintaining clear vision and relative comfort throughout their lives. Further research to identify more completely the pathogenetic mechanisms involved in development of the dry eye is ongoing. It is hoped that the results of such studies will allow us to direct our therapies more specifically and even more successfully in the near future.

■ References

1. Holly FJ, Lemp MA. Tear physiology and dry eyes. Surv Ophthalmol 1977;22(2):69–87
2. Dart DA. Physiology of tear production. In: Lemp MA, Marquardt R, eds. The dry eye: a comprehensive guide. New York: Springer-Verlag, 1992
3. Kramer PW, York KK, Lubkin V, et al. Tamoxifen effect on the rabbit lacrimal gland and ocular mucous glycoprotein. Invest Ophthalmol Vis Sci 1984;25:191
4. Jacobs M, Buxton D, Kramer P, et al. The effect of oophorectomy on the rabbit lacrimal system. Invest Ophthalmol Vis Sci 1986;27:25
5. Kramer P, Lubken V, Potter W. Cyclical changes in conjunctival smears from menstruating females. Ophthalmology 1990;97:303–307
6. Wilson SE. Lacrimal epidermal growth factor production and the ocular surface. Am J Ophthalmol 1991;111:763–765
7. Mathers WP, Shields WJ, Sachdev MS, et al. Meibomian gland dysfunction in chronic blepharitis. Cornea 1991;10:277–285
8. Lemp MA. Artificial tear solutions in the tear film and dry eye syndromes. Int Ophthalmol Clin 1973;13(1):221–229
9. Katz JI, Kaufman HE, Breslin C, Katz IM. Slow release artificial tears and the treatment of keratitis sicca. Ophthalmology 1978;86:787–793

10. Lamberts DW, Langston DP, Chu W. A clinical study of slow-releasing artificial tears. Ophthalmology 1978;85:794–800
11. Benson DR, Hemmady PB, Snyder RW. Efficacy of laser punctal occlusion. Ophthalmol 1992;99:618–621
12. Rolando R, Refojo MF, Kenyon KR. Increased tear film evaporation in eyes with keratoconjunctivitis sicca. Arch Ophthalmol 1983;101:557–558
13. Foster CS, Watson LA, Ekins MB. Immunosuppressive therapy for progressive ocular cicatricial pemphigoid. Ophthalmology 1982;89:340–352
14. John T, Refojo MF, Hannineu L, et al. Cornea 1989;8(1):21–31
15. Tseng SCG, Maumenee AE, Stark WJ, et al. Topical retinoid treatment for various dry-eye disorders. Ophthalmol 1985;92:917–927
16. Lubkin V. Drugs for topical applications of sex steroid in the treatment of dry eye syndrome and methods of preparations and application: US Patent 5,041,434. August 20, 1991
17. Bennett JE. The management of total xerophthalmia. Arch Ophthalmol 1969;81:667–682
18. American Academy of Ophthalmology. Basic and clinical science course. Sec 7 1990–91:270
19. Lemp MA. General measures in management of the dry eye. Int Ophthalmol Clin 1987;27(1):36–43

New Approaches to Dry-Eye Therapy

Kazuo Tsubota, M.D.

Although the definitive cure remains elusive, dry eye can often be successfully controlled with available therapies, including artificial tears, lacrimal punctal plugs, and treatment of accompanying diseases such as meibomianitis and allergic conjunctivitis. Dry eye is the subject of intense active research, which has provided greater insight into the condition along with new approaches to its management.

This chapter reviews four new approaches to dry-eye treatment (Fig 1). First, the prevention of tear evaporation is an old but important technique [1], which often alleviates symptoms in certain dry-eye patients. Several new studies have identified factors that predispose to tear evaporation, along with some techniques to minimize it. Second, research on artificial tears is now focused on the mechanisms of tear stability on the ocular surface rather than simply the maintenance of a certain tear volume. Recent studies have shown that the mucin layer is more critical to maintaining tear integrity than was previously believed [2, 3]. Third, such drugs as epidermal growth factor (EGF) [4] and aldose reductase inhibitors (ARI) [5], although not direct treatments for dry eye, do help to protect the corneal epithelium. Fourth, there is considerable interest in the immunological aspects of dry eye. Tear deficiency alone cannot explain all the cases of dry eye, and we believe that direct involvement of the ocular surface is the underlying cause of many cases of dry eye [6, 7]. Immune-targeted eye drops can modify the lymphocytic activities in the conjunctiva and lacrimal gland. Indeed, cyclosporine A has been reported to be effective for the treatment of canine dry eye [8] and may also be effective for certain types of dry eye in humans.

■ Tear Evaporation

Tear production under normal circumstances is reported by Mishima and coworkers [9] to be 1.2 µl/min and by Scherz and colleagues [10] to

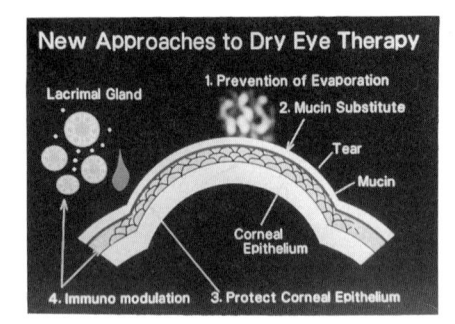

Figure 1 New approaches to dry-eye therapy: (1) prevention of tear evaporation, (2) new artificial tears as mucin substitute, (3) corneal epithelial protection, and (4) immune-targeted eye drops.

be 0.6 to 1.1 μl/min, whereas tear evaporation is reported to be 26.9 × 10^{-7} gm/sec by Hamano and associates [11], 4.1 × 10^{-7} gm/sec by Rolando's group [12], and 15.6 × 10^{-7} gm/sec (0.094 μl/min) by Tsubota and coworkers [13]. Combining Mishima's and Tsubota's data indicates that tear evaporation is 7.8% of production. However, dry eye often is associated with diminished tear production, Schirmer's test values being as low as 1 mm or less (compared with a normal result of at least 10 mm). If the absolute tear evaporation in such cases does not decrease, then it represents at least 78% of tear loss (Fig 2). Even if evaporation decreases to 9.5 × 10^{-7} gm/sec (0.057 μl/min) in dry eyes, as we have reported [13], 47.5% of tear production (much more than normal) still is being lost to evaporation.

It is often noted that dry-eye patients suffer more under windy or dry conditions, which accelerate tear evaporation. Users of video display terminals (VDT) also often complain of ocular fatigue, irritation, and a feeling of heaviness. The major symptom of dry eye is ocular fatigue [14], and recent work has shown that VDT workers tend to experience accelerated tear evaporation and, hence, dry-eye symptoms as a result of decreased blink rate and increased palpebral fissures [15].

Blink Rate and Exposed Ocular Surface Area

Blinking is essential for inducing tear secretion and spreading the aqueous, mucin, and lipid layers over the cornea [16]. Between blinks, the tear film thins as a result of evaporation and drainage, exposing a bare cornea if the interval is too great [17]. In a study of 104 healthy office workers (45 men and 59 women; age range 20 to 69 years), at 22.5°C and 40% humidity, blink rate averaged 22 ± 9 per minute under relaxed conditions, 10 ± 6 per minute while the subjects were reading a book at table level, and 7 ± 7 per minute while the subjects were viewing text on a VDT [15]. The corresponding exposed ocular surface areas, calculated by measuring the palpebral fissure width, were 2.2 ± 0.4 cm², 1.2 ± 0.4 cm², and 2.3 ± 0.5 cm², respectively. Not only did tear evaporation in-

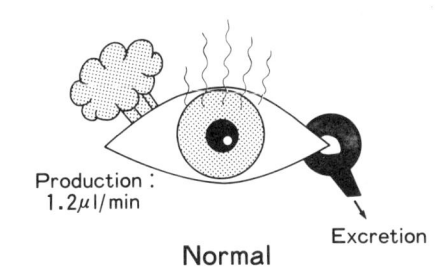

New Dry-Eye Therapy ■ 117

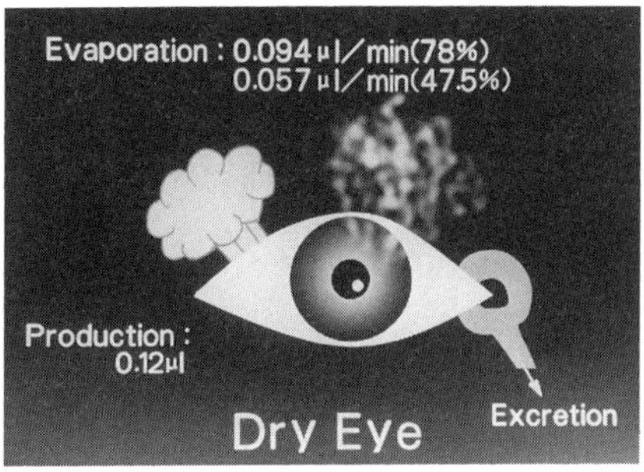

Figure 2 *(A) In the normal eye, tear evaporation is less than 10% of total tear loss. (B) In the dry eye, tear evaporation represents 47.5 to 78% of total tear loss.*

crease along with exposed ocular surface area, but the evaporation rate per unit area also increased, suggesting a qualitative instability of the tear film over larger surfaces (Fig 3A).

Of course, any activity or occupation that requires particular visual concentration predisposes individuals to developing ocular fatigue and other dry-eye symptoms. Takano and associates [18] reported that the interval between blinks for ophthalmologists under normal circumstances is 2.1 ± 0.4 seconds, but increases to 3.7 ± 2.6 during biomicroscopy, 4.3 ± 2.2 during tonometry, and 4.8 ± 2.0 while performing a fundus examination. Surgical procedures substantially increase this interval further to 10.5 ± 4.2 seconds during photocoagulation and 30.5 ± 27.9 seconds during cataract surgery [18]. Certain ergonomic modifications, such as placing VDTs at a lower level so that workers do not have to keep their eyes so open, may alleviate some of these symptoms (Fig 3B, C). Instructing people to blink intentionally also may help, as may the use of a room humidifier. As described next, we have developed another technique for dealing with dry eyes that, for whatever reason, remains refractory to simpler measures.

Moisture Glasses

Tear evaporation depends on the environmental humidity: It is maximal at an ambient humidity of 0% and decreases to 0 at 100% humidity.

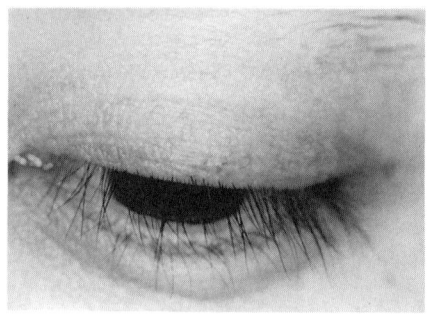

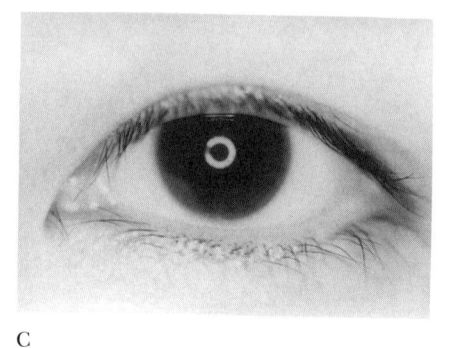

Figure 3 (A) Tear evaporation and ocular surface area, which depend on the eye position. (B, C) Ocular surface area affected by reading (B) and video display terminal work (C). When patients look down, the palpebral fissure and ocular surface area are smallest, resulting in the least tear evaporation.

We have devised special glasses that employ wet sponges inserted on side panels to increase the humidity surrounding the eyes (Fig 4) [19]. The side panels serve both to hold the sponges and to act as additional barriers to evaporative loss. Figure 5 shows the humidity near the cornea in a typical dry-eye patient. Humidity is highest using the glasses with sponges and side panels, and lowest with spectacles, frame only (no lenses). In a clinical trial of 16 patients using moisture glasses, all reported greater comfort and showed objective improvement [19].

For daily use, a simple therapeutic regimen is necessary. Although swimming goggles or plastic sheets can keep moisture levels high, they are uncomfortable and aesthetically unappealing. Moisture glasses are considered to be a desirable alternative, providing steady evaporation of water from the sponge to maintain the high humidity level. The sponges are replaced every 1 to 2 weeks, and the side panels also are replaceable.

■ New Artificial Tears

Several new artificial tear preparations are in various stages of development. All are preservative-free and contain viscoelastic materials, the latter taking on greater significance with the realization of the role of the mucin

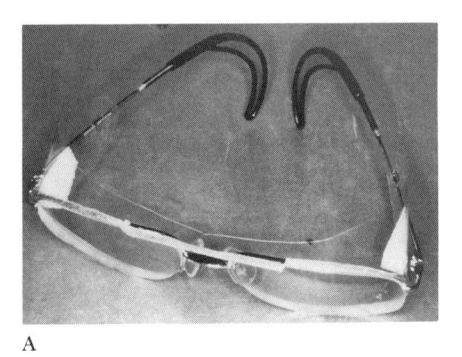

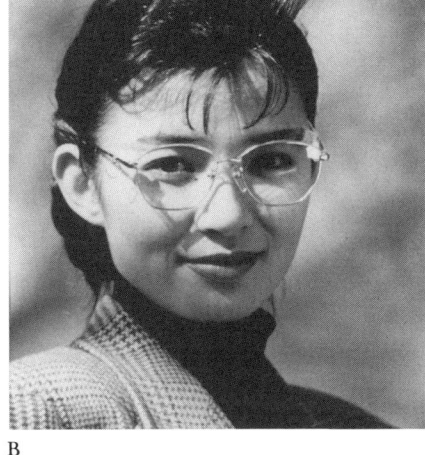

Figure 4 (A, B) Moisture glasses, in which side panels with moist sponges are attached to the frame.

layer in maintaining tear film integrity. The following three drops are currently used in our clinic.

Hyaluronic Acid

Hyaluronic acid is well-established in cataract surgery and penetrating keratoplasty for the prevention of endothelial damage. Although it has been used to treat dry eye for several years [20, 21], a multicenter study concluded that it does not affect the conjunctiva as determined by impression cytology [22], so that the efficacy of hyaluronic acid for the treatment of dry eye remains controversial. We performed a double-blind multicenter study using 0.1% hyaluronic acid for the treatment of 104 dry-eye patients and found significant improvement in corneal fluorescein but not rose bengal staining in patients treated with hyaluronic acid compared with those who received a placebo [23].

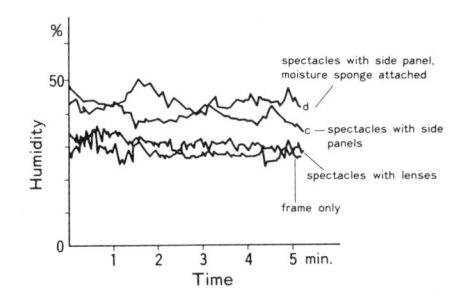

Figure 5 Ambient humidity level above the cornea with various types of spectacles.

It has been reported that hyaluronic acid is effective in the wound healing of the corneal epithelium [24]. The use of hyaluronic acid for corneal ulcers has been examined in a multicenter study in Japan, with enhanced healing of persistent epithelial defects (Fig 6). Hyaluronic acid seems to be beneficial not only as a mucin substitute but also as a fibronectin inducer in dry-eye management.

RGD Peptide

RGD consists of three amino acids—arginine, glycine, and aspartate—that form the binding site for fibronectin and other RGD-containing ligand for integrin, which is the surface glycoprotein for mediating cellular adhesion. In wound healing, the RGD binding site is necessary for epithelial cell attachment to and movement on the cornea.

We have had some success treating dry eye with a new artificial tear compound containing 18 peptides with the RGD sequence, combined with chondroitin sulfate. One patient was a 38-year-old man with simple dry eye and superior limbic keratitis who used drops containing RGD peptide and chondroitin sulfate for 1 month. Rose bengal staining of the superior limbic portion of the eye was greatly improved.

Both the RGD and chondroitin sulfate portions can mediate adhesion to the corneal epithelium, acting as mucin and prolonging the tear film breakup time. These drops may also prevent bacterial adhesion to the epithelium. It is speculated that *Pseudomonas aeruginosa* uses RGD sequence for its adhesion to cells. Our preliminary study has shown that a medium with RGD in a concentration of 0.1 mg/ml successfully prevented the adhesion of *P. aeruginosa* in a culture dish. Dry eye is a risk factor for ulcerative keratitis, especially in patients who wear contact lenses. RGD peptide drops may thus serve to diminish both dryness and infection, although further clinical evaluation is necessary.

High-Viscosity Methylcellulose

According to Feenstra and Tseng [25], rose bengal stains epithelium uncovered by mucin or other viscous proteins, and methylcellulose has been shown to prevent rose bengal staining in vitro. Low-concentration methylcellulose is a well-established viscoelastic material in artificial tears [26]; recently, drops containing very high concentration methylcellulose (hydroxypropyl methylcellulose) have been introduced (Visco Tears, Alcon Laboratory, Fort Worth, TX). We used very high-viscosity methylcellulose drops for the treatment of dry eye in Sjögren's syndrome and found decreased rose bengal as well as fluorescein staining (Fig 7), although patients with only mild to moderate symptoms disliked the high-viscosity preparation.

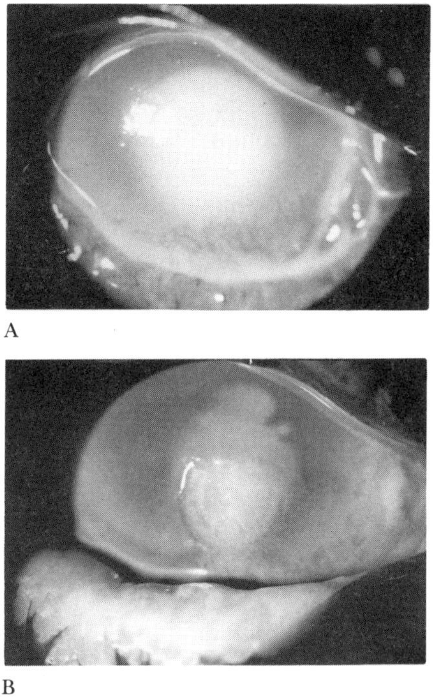

New Dry-Eye Therapy ■ 121

Figure 6 *(A) Persistent epithelial defect. (B) Two weeks after treatment with 0.1% hyaluronic acid, the epithelial defect is healed.*

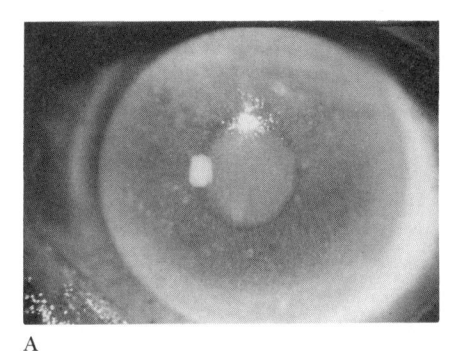

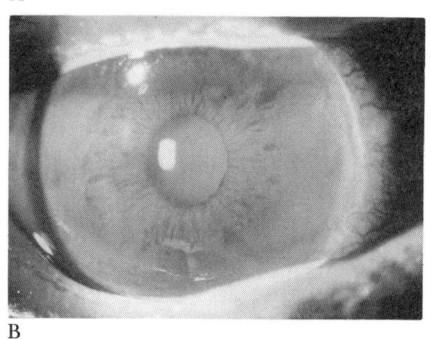

Figure 7 *Treatment of Sjögren's syndrome by high-viscosity methylcellulose. (A) Rose bengal and fluorescein staining of the ocular surface were persistent. (B) After application of high-concentration methylcellulose, the staining decreased along with a decrease in subjective complaints.*

Corneal Epithelium

Although dry eye is caused by abnormal tear production, loss, or composition, it may be exacerbated by or, in turn, exacerbate disorders of the corneal epithelium. When the epithelium is compromised, management of dry eye is difficult, and so treatments for the epithelium can complement those for dry eye.

Epidermal Growth Factor

EGF is present in tears and may play a role in the normal maintenance and wound healing of the corneal epithelium [27]. Because dry-eye patients have a paucity of tears, the epithelium may receive insufficient EGF. The use of EGF in dry-eye patients is now under investigation, but preliminary results are not promising. It may be that EGF can be provided from the stromal side and that supplemental EGF in tears may not improve the epithelium in dry eye.

Nevertheless, EGF may strengthen the ocular surface epithelium [4]. The use of EGF in Sjögren's syndrome patients who lack reflex tearing is also currently under investigation [28].

Aldose Reductase Inhibitor

In diabetes, tear dynamics often are abnormal, possibly due to decreased sensitivity of the ocular surface [29]. Aldose reductase is activated to produce excess sorbitol which, because it cannot pass through the cell wall, accumulates inside and interferes with cell function. This is the primary mechanism of diabetic changes in the neurons and the crystalline lens. Although diabetic patients typically have epithelial staining by fluorescein, they do not complain as much as ordinary dry-eye patients, probably because of their decreased sensitivity [29]. We have found that the corneal epithelial morphological changes in diabetic patients [30] can be reversed by topical ARI (0.25% of CT112; Senju Pharmaceutical, Osaka, Japan) (Fig 8) [31], although currently only an oral formulation of ARI (Kinedak, Ono Pharmaceuticals, Osaka, Japan) is commercially available in Japan.

Vitamin A

Vitamin A is provided to the corneal epithelium by tears [32], so a deficiency is expected in certain cases of dry eye, especially Sjögren's syndrome. Retinoic acid is a major form of vitamin A, and retinol can be metabolized to retinoic acid [33, 34]. We obtained promising results with artificial tears containing retinol, 500 IU/ml; brush cytology showed a decrease in keratinized cells (Fig 9). Because we did not achieve similar suc-

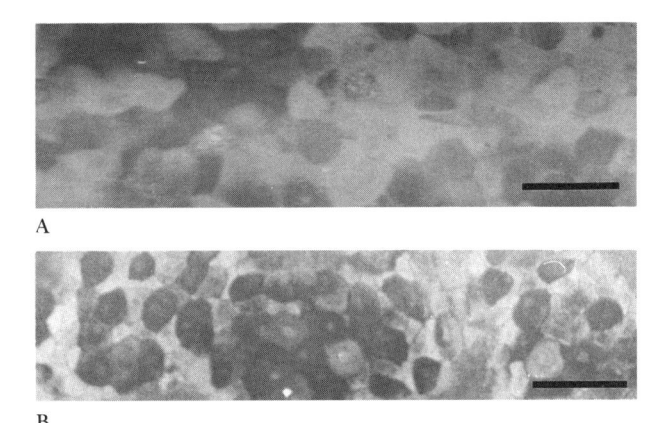

Figure 8 Corneal epithelium in diabetic patients as observed by specular microscopy. (A) Before treatment, the epithelial cell size is large. (B) After application of topical aldose reductase inhibitor, the cell size returned to normal.

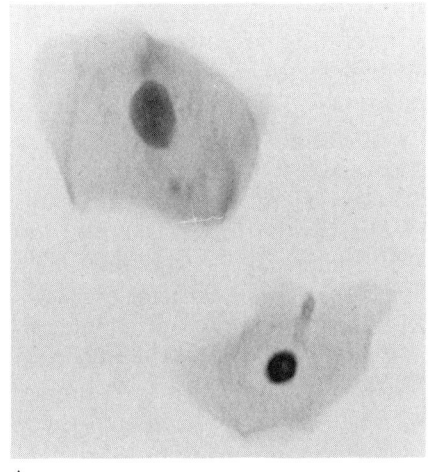

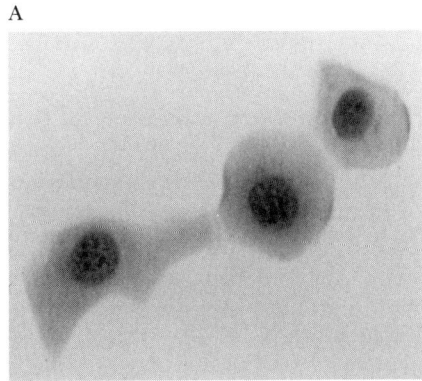

Figure 9 Conjunctival epithelial cells in Sjögren's syndrome, treated with vitamin A. Keratinized cells are observed before treatment (A) but decrease after vitamin A application (B).

cess with this regimen in non-Sjögren's dry eye, it may be that occasional reflex tearing can supply the vitamin A to the corneal epithelium in non-Sjögren's cases. A more comprehensive clinical trial employing brush cytology is now under way to evaluate vitamin A treatment for dry eye; results are due in the spring of 1994.

Immunotherapy

Although the primary mechanism of dry eye is a qualitative or quantitative defect in the tear film layers, some types of dry eye are caused by immunological disorders, such as lymphocyte infiltration into the lacrimal gland and conjunctiva in Sjögren's syndrome. In such cases, modulation of the underlying immune response may prove more efficacious than the frequent use of artificial tears.

Cyclosporine A

Recently, my colleagues and I reported that granzyme A and perforin mediate lacrimal gland destruction by cytolytic T cells [35]. Cytolytic T-cell function can be suppressed with cyclosporine A or FK506 following kidney transplantation, and similar immunological modulation is being investigated to treat Sjögren's syndrome. Cyclosporine A is a potent drug capable of suppressing the cytolytic T lymphocyte [36], and it has shown promise in vitro and in the treatment of canine dry eye [8]. Clinical application has been complicated by the difficulty in developing a suitable vehicle for topical use. Peanut oils have been used for several years but cause ocular irritation. Recently, cyclodextran was proposed as a medium in which cyclosporine A (0.05%) can be dissolved, and we are now successfully using this formulation [37]. Preliminary clinical results are encouraging, with favorable subjective and objective patient response (Fig 10). A multicenter trial will soon be conducted in Japan.

Interferon-α

Epstein-Barr virus (EBV) is believed to be associated with the development of Sjögren's syndrome [38–40], and so investigations of the use of interferon-α drops for the treatment of dry eye in Sjögren's syndrome are ongoing [40–42]. Preliminary results show that concentrations as low as 20 units/ml can suppress EBV in vitro. Concentrations of up to 2 million units/ml, used four to five times daily, are being tested in clinical trials. Approximately half the patients reported subjective improvement with fewer EBV genomes in superficial conjunctival cells obtained by brush cytology (Fig 11). An optimal dosing regimen remains to be determined, but interferon-α appears to have a place in the treatment of certain types of dry eye.

New Dry-Eye Therapy ■ 125

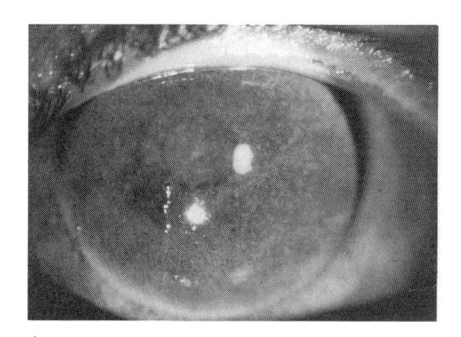

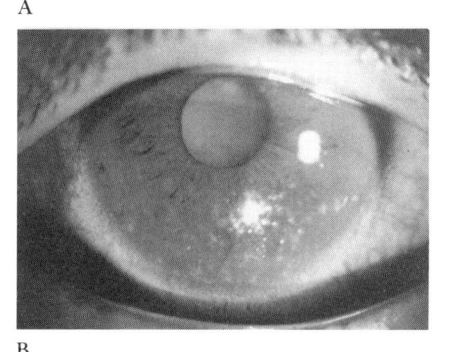

Figure 10 Rose bengal and fluorescein staining of ocular surface in Sjögren's syndrome patients (A) before and (B) after cyclosporine A application. Vital staining decreased after 1 month of cyclosporine A use.

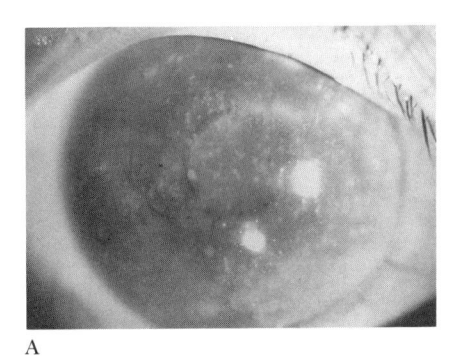

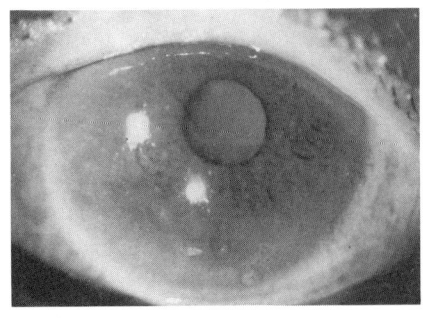

Figure 11 Rose bengal and fluorescein staining of the ocular surface in Sjögren's syndrome patients (A) before and (B) after use of interferon alpha. Vital staining and subjective complaints decreased 2 months after treatment. This patient had prolonged improvement even after cessation of the treatment.

■ Conclusion

There are several new approaches to dry-eye therapy based on concepts detailed in this chapter. In addition to the widely accepted treatments of punctal occlusion and frequent application of artificial tears, the prevention of evaporation is very important and effective. Moisture glasses, intentional blinking, and environmental modification are relatively simple measures that entail no side effects.

The mucin layer is critical in stabilizing tears; a defect in it typically leads to dry-eye symptoms and may cause some cases of contact lens intolerance. New artificial tears are increasingly formulated as mucin substitutes or as direct treatments for the epithelium (e.g., EGF).

One of the most promising new treatments for dry eye is immunotherapy, which offers the possibility of directly treating the underlying pathology in certain cases. Considerable research is being done to understand local or systemic defects in the immune system at the molecular level. I believe that a combination of these and other new approaches will increasingly provide dramatic relief to chronic sufferers of the often debilitating condition of dry eye.

■ References

1. Tsubota K. The effect of wearing spectacles on the humidity of the eye. Am J Ophthalmol 1989;108:92–93
2. Prydal J, Campbell F. Study of precorneal tear film thickness and structure by interferometry and confocal microscopy. Invest Ophthalmol Vis Sci 1992;33:1996–2005
3. Prydal J, Artal P, Woon H, Campbell F. Study of human precorneal tear film thickness and structure using laser interferometry. Invest Ophthalmol Vis Sci 1992;33:2006–2011
4. Mathers W, Sherman M, Fryczkowski A, Jester J. Dose-dependent effects of epidermal growth factor on corneal wound healing. Invest Ophthalmol Vis Sci 1989;30:2403–2406
5. Ohashi Y, Matsuda M, Kinoshita S, Manabe R. Aldose reductase inhibitor (CT-112) eyedrops for diabetic corneal epitheliopathy. Am J Ophthalmol 1988;105:233–238
6. Pflugfelder S, Huang A, Feuer W, et al. Conjunctival cytologic features of primary Sjögren's syndrome. Ophthalmology 1990;97:985–993
7. Hikichi T, Yoshida A, Tsubota K. Lymphocytic infiltration of the conjunctiva and the salivary gland in Sjögren's syndrome. Arch Ophthalmol 1993;111:21–22
8. Kaswan RL, Salisbury MA, Ward DA. Spontaneous canine keratoconjunctivitis sicca. A useful model for human keratoconjunctivitis sicca: treatment with cyclosporine eye drops. Arch Ophthalmol 1989;107:1210–1216
9. Mishima S, Gasset A, Klyce S, Baum J. Determination of tear volume and tear flow. Invest Ophthalmol Vis Sci 1966;5:264–276
10. Scherz W, Doane M, Dohlman C. Tear volume in normal eyes and keratoconjunctivitis sicca. Albrecht von Graefes Arch Klin Exp Ophthalmol 1974;192:141–150
11. Hamano H, Hori M, Mitsunaga S. Application of the evaporimeter to the ophthalmic field. J Jpn Cl Soc 1990;22:101–107

12. Rolando M, Refojo M. Tear evaporimeter for measuring water evaporation rate from the tear film under controlled conditions in humans. Exp Eye Res 1983;36: 25–33
13. Tsubota K, Yamada M. Tear evaporation from the ocular surface. Invest Ophthalmol Vis Sci 1992;33:2942–2950
14. Toda I, Fujishima H, Tsubota K. Ocular fatigue is the major symptom of dry eye. Acta Ophthalmol (Copenh) 1993;71:347–352
15. Tsubota K, Nakamori K. Dry eyes and video display terminals. N Engl J Med 1993;328:584
16. Holly F. Physical chemistry of the normal and disordered tear film. Trans Ophthalmol Soc UK 1985;104:374–378
17. Holly F. Formation and rupture of the tear film. Exp Eye Res 1973;15:515–525
18. Takano H, Takamura E, Yoshino K, Tsubota K. The increase of the blink interval in ophthalmic procedures. In: Proceedings of The First International Congress of Lacrimal Gland, Tear and Dry Eye. 1994:in press
19. Tsubota K, Yamada M, Urayama K. Spectacle side panels and moist inserts for the treatment of dry eye patients. Cornea 1994:in press
20. Limberg M, McCae C, Kissling H, Kaufman H. Topical application of hyaluronic acid and chondroitin sulfate in the treatment of dry eyes. Am J Ophthalmol 1987; 103:194–197
21. Sand B, Marner K, Norn M. Sodium hyaluronate in the treatment of keratoconjunctivitis sicca. A double masked clinical trial. Acta Ophthalmol (Copenh) 1989;67: 181–183
22. Nelson J, Farris R. Sodium hyaluronate and polyvinyl alcohol artificial tear preparations. Arch Ophthalmol 1988;106:484–487
23. Shimmura S, Mashima Y, Shimazaki J, et al. The effect of sodium hyaluronate ophthalmic solution on dry eye. J Eye 1993;10:611–616
24. Nishida T, Nakamura M, Mishima H, Otori T. Hyaluronan stimulates corneal epithelial migration. Exp Eye Res 1991;53:753–758
25. Feenstra R, Tseng S. What is actually stained by rose bengal? Arch Ophthalmol 1992;110:984–993
26. Bron A. Prospects for the dry eye (Duke-Elder lecture). Trans Ophthalmol Soc UK 1985;104:801–826
27. Ohashi Y, Motokura M, Kinoshita Y, et al. Presence of epidermal growth factor in human tears. Invest Ophthalmol Vis Sci 1989;30:1879–1887
28. Tsubota K. The importance of the Schirmer test with nasal stimulation [lett]. Am J Ophthalmol 1991;111:106–108
29. Ogawa Y, Kamoshita I, Yoshino K, et al. Dry eye in diabetics. J Eye 1992;9: 1867–1870
30. Tsubota K, Chiba K, Shimazaki J. Corneal epithelium in diabetic patients. Cornea 1991;10:156–160
31. Tsubota K, Yamada M. The effect of aldose reductase inhibitor on the corneal epithelium. Cornea 1993;12:161–162
32. Ubels JL, Loley K, Rismondo V. Retinol secretion by the lacrimal gland. Invest Ophthalmol Vis Sci 1986;27:1261–1269
33. Ubels JL, Edelhauser HF. In vivo metabolism of topically applied retinol and all-trans retinoic acid by the rabbit cornea. Biochem Biophys Res Commun 1985;131: 320–327
34. Rask L, Geijer C, Bill A, Peterson PA. Vitamin A supply of the cornea. Exp Eye Res 1980;31:201–211
35. Tsubota K, Saito I, Miyasaka N. Detection of granzyme A and perforin in lacrimal gland of Sjögren's syndrome. Am J Ophthalmol 1994:in press
36. O'Keefe S, Tamura J, Kincaid R, et al. FK-506 and CsA-sensitive activation of the interleukin-2 promoter by calcineurin. Nature 1992;357:692–694

37. Kanai A, Alba RM, Takano T, et al. The effect on the cornea of alpha cyclodextrin vehicle for cyclosporin eye drops. Transplant Proc 1989;21:3150–3152
38. Pflugfelder SC, Crouse C, Pereira I, Atherton S. Amplification of Epstein-Barr virus genomic sequences in blood cells, lacrimal glands, and tears from primary Sjögren's syndrome patients. Ophthalmology 1990;97:976–984
39. Saito I, Servenius B, Compton T, Fox R. Detection of Epstein-Barr virus DNA by polymerase chain reaction in blood and tissue biopsies from patients with Sjögren's syndrome. J Exp Med 1989;169:2191–2198
40. Pflugfelder SC, Roussel T, Culbertson W. Primary Sjögren's syndrome after infectious mononucleosis. JAMA 1987;257:1049–1050
41. Lotz M, Tsoukas C, Fong S, et al. Regulation of Epstein-Barr virus infection by recombinant interferons. Selected sensitivity to interferon-gamma. Eur J Immunol 1985;15:520–525
42. Kumar R, Atlas I. Interferon alpha induces the expression of retinoblastoma gene product in human Burkitt lymphoma Daudi cells: role in growth regulation. Proc Natl Acad Sci USA 1992;89:6599–6603
43. Kure S, Tada K, Wada J, Yoshie O. Inhibition of Epstein-Barr virus infection in vitro by recombinant human interferon alpha and gamma. Virus Res 1986;5:377–390

Contact Lenses and the Dry Eye

R. Linsy Farris, M.D.

Contact lens fitters commonly hear the claim that an individual cannot wear contact lenses because he or she has dry eyes, which immediately raises two questions: Does this person really have dry eyes and, if so, how severe is the dry-eye condition? The answers to these questions will determine whether another trial with contact lenses is likely to achieve favorable results.

Because contact lens wear as a treatment for dry eyes is unproved at the present time, I am concerned in this chapter with the clinical detection and diagnosis of the dry eye in individuals who wish to wear contact lenses or in those already wearing contact lenses but to only a limited degree and with considerable discomfort. Reviewed in this chapter are methods of evaluating a contact lens wearer for the presence and severity of a dry-eye condition, the multiple mechanisms of tear film abnormality that may be responsible for contact lens intolerance and, finally, the range of therapies available to improve and relieve the dry eye during contact lens wear.

■ Dry Eye, Blepharitis, and Allergic Conjunctivitis

The diagnosis of dry eye (see the chapter by Dr Nelson in this issue) requires close attention in the patient who has been told he or she has dry eyes and cannot wear contact lenses. Clinical examination will yield subtle clues such as a deficient inferior marginal tear strip, excessive debris in the tear film, and a viscous or hypofluorescent tear film in the dry-eye patient. More important, however, than these signs is the ability of the resting-state tears to produce reflex tears as measured by Schirmer's test without anesthetic. Wetting of more than 5 mm of the Schirmer strip in 5 minutes reassures one that the lacrimal gland is normal in its ability to produce tears on demand, such as is required when contact lenses become dry as a result of increased tear evaporation [1].

Blepharitis is frequently detected in the clinical examination and provides an additional explanation for dry eyes in the failed contact lens wearer. Inadequate meibomian oils may be a contributing mechanism to poor tear function by failing to provide constituents for the oily layer on the surface of the tear film that are required to prevent tear evaporation [2]. Blepharitis frequently is overlooked, particularly when it is of such a mild degree that the only evidence is occlusion of the meibomian gland openings. Gentle pressure on the lower eyelids serves as a test in determining the percentage of meibomian glands that are occluded and therefore not contributing secretions to the tear film. Fair-skinned individuals are more likely to have meibomian gland occlusion and more severe forms of blepharitis, characterized by erythema, large plugs of keratin that elevate from the eyelid margin, or concretions on the lashes. The treatment is application of warm tap-water compresses on the closed eyelids for 1 minute twice daily after face washing, followed by wiping of the lower eyelid margin with a tightly wound cotton-tipped applicator while viewing in a mirror [3]. For most individuals, the latter maneuver is too difficult for the upper eyelids but can be managed for the lower lid margins, which have more mucus and oils than do the upper lids. The treatment should be demonstrated with the patient observing in a hand mirror and is explained as being similar to cleaning a window ledge. The technique, which provides daily massage of the meibomian orifices as well as removal of keratin plugs, excess mucus and oils, is simple and cheap, thus ensuring long-term compliance. Such attention to the lower eyelid margin removes materials that gain access to the tear film through the inferior marginal tear strip, interfere with the tears' ability to moisten the cornea, and contaminate the surfaces of contact lenses.

The upper tarsal conjunctiva provides important information regarding the sensitivity of ocular tissues in patients who have eyes that react adversely to contact lens wear and environmental pollutants. These individuals may have received a diagnosis of dry eyes and indeed may have dry eyes as a result of excessive tear evaporation, but they also may have allergic conjunctivitis. Giant papillary conjunctivitis is a well-known and easily recognized entity arising from chronic exposure of the upper palpebral conjunctiva to plastic in prostheses, contact lenses, and exposed nylon suture tips [4].

A milder form of upper tarsal conjunctiva reaction is apparent in many allergy-prone individuals and contact lens wearers who complain of eye discomfort and itching. The upper tarsal conjunctiva demonstrates small elevations less than 1.0 mm in diameter that are widely spaced and usually in a red background. These contact lens wearers appear to have a mild form of allergic conjunctivitis. I grade such a reaction as trace to 4+ and label it *folliculosis*. Symptoms usually are relieved by preservative-free artificial tears and a preservative-free lens care regimen. New soft contact lenses usually are required as deposits form on the contact lens immediately during wear and these deposits, as well as the contact lens matrix, tend to lock in preservatives from lens care systems. As a result, the lens produces a continuous antigenic stimulus during contact lens wear and a localized allergic reaction in the upper tarsal conjunctiva [5]. Disposable contact lenses have provided an even more effective means of improving these symptoms of allergic conjunctivitis and dry eye during contact lens wear, by avoiding the buildup of deposits containing preservatives from lens solution [6].

■ Dry-Eye Mechanisms

When a dry eye is diagnosed in the presence of adequate reflex tearing, as can occur in contact lens wearers, one must consider the primary mechanisms responsible for tear film integrity. A review of the five primary mechanisms responsible for tear film maintenance can determine whether contact lenses are detrimental or beneficial in the maintenance of an adequate tear film. *Lambs* is a mnemonic device that may help one recall the five mechanisms of tear film maintenance [3].

Lipid Abnormality

A disturbance of lipids in the tear film may be the most frequently encountered contact lens–related tear film disturbance. A greasy appearance of the anterior contact lens surface is extremely common and often is the cause of blurred vision. The eyelid margins have excessive mucous debris and oils. The meibomian gland orifices contain firm yellow plugs that may be expressed by gentle pressure on the eyelid margin. Teenagers are most frequently bothered by this problem, although older individuals are also affected owing to neglect of the eyelid margins during face washing. Lipids in the tear film and from the eyelid margins diffuse into the tear film and through the mucin layer to the epithelial surface. Contamination of the mucin layer with lipid has been proposed as a method of dry-spot formation [7].

Aqueous Abnormality

Total tear volume averages 7.0 + 2.0 μl, with 1.1 + 0.02 μl in the precorneal tear film, 2.9 μl in the marginal tear meniscus, and 4.5 μl in the cul-de-sac [8, 9]. The volume of tears beneath a contact lens is approximately 2 μl, and there is a normal turnover rate of approximately 20% on each blink in a well-adapted hard corneal contact lens wearer [10]. The dry eye resulting from a tear volume abnormality demonstrates not only decreased tear flow but also lower tear volume [8]. Reduced tear volume and tear flow in a contact lens wearer with a dry eye decreases the movement of a contact lens, which produces a tight appearance on slit-lamp examination. Manipulation of the eyelids and the contact lens may produce an adequate stimulus for reflex tearing so that, very quickly, the dry appearance may change to one of excessive tears. Tear film status can be assessed via examination of the inferior marginal tear strip through the slit lamp using only overhead illumination and no illumination from within the lamp itself, as illumination from the slit lamp provokes reflex tearing, artifactual excessive lens movement, and an enlarged inferior marginal tear strip.

Mucin Abnormality

Lemp and coworkers [11] first brought to our attention causes of dry eye other than volume deficiency. They demonstrated that mucin substances are necessary to permit spreading of the tears across the cornea by decreasing the contact angle of tear droplets. Tear film breakup time was developed as a clinical measurement of the ability of tears to moisten the corneal surface. Although these investigators pointed to a mucin deficiency in certain dry-eye states, others noted excessive mucin strands in the dry eye [12, 13]. We now understand that there are two types of mucin present in tears, an invisible mucin that dissolves in tears [14] and a visible form that represents degraded mucin, which is of lesser benefit in promoting wetting of the ocular surface [13]. In contact lens wearers with an abnormal mucin layer, excess mucin debris and increased epithelial staining could occur because of excessive degradation of tear mucins and decreased tear film wetting of the corneal surface. Holly [15, 16] has stressed the importance of tear mucins and the mucin layer in contact lens wear.

Treatment of mucin abnormalities in the contact lens wearer consists of increasing hydration and removing mucin strands by cleaning the contact lenses more frequently. Acetylcysteine has been used as an eye drop to improve mucin liquefaction. Sodium hyaluronate is potentially useful as an artificial mucin because its structure traps water and facilitates adhesion to cell surfaces [17]. Attempts have been made to use tear film breakup time as a test of mucin deficiency, but the variability and brevity of this phenomenon in normal subjects has limited its usefulness in the evaluation of dry eyes [18, 19].

Base Abnormality

Several disorders are associated with abnormalities of the corneal epithelium that forms a base for the tear film. Bandage contact lenses have been used therapeutically in many patients to provide increased comfort and improved vision [20]. In cases of recurrent erosion and persistent epithelial defects, the soft therapeutic bandage contact lens serves as a protective covering and encourages reepithelialization of the cornea.

Surface Abnormality

Blinking in the contact lens wearer is important not only to spread the tear film across the corneal and conjunctival surface but also to produce lens movement and exchange of tears beneath the contact lens. In addition to preventing hypoxia, tear exchange is helpful in preventing a buildup of epithelial debris from shedding surface cells beneath the lens. Studies have indicated the hypertonic tear film in the dry-eye patient increases the rate of epithelial degeneration [21]. An increased rate of epithelial exfoliation would also be more likely in a dry-eye patient because anoxia may develop as a result of decreased tear exchange owing to decreased tear volume.

Contact lens wear interferes with the spreading of the tear film across the corneal surface by the eyelids. At the contact lens edges, where minimal movement occurs, a pool of tears develops beneath the eyelid margin, resulting in 3- and 9-o'clock staining [22]. Diffuse corneal staining also is more likely to occur as a result of the increased rate of epithelial surface cell desquamation seen in both contact lens wear and the dry eye. Scanning electron microscopical studies have revealed flattening of surface reticulation and cellular desquamation consequent to rigid methylmethacrylate and soft contact lens wear. In contrast, in wearers of ultrathin hydrogel lenses with greater gas permeability, there was no evidence of surface ultrastructural alteration [23].

■ Contact Lens Wear as a Cause of Dry Eye

Contact lens wear may cause at least a mild degree of dry eye, such that the patient may complain of symptoms similar to those of dry eye and the signs of tear film disturbance similar to those observed in dry-eye patients may be produced [1]. Subjectively, contact lens wearers have found that the use of artificial tear drops, or so-called comfort drops, relieve eye irritation associated with contact lens wear. They also have discovered that environmental conditions, particularly wind or air conditioning, often are responsible for greater discomfort with contact lens wear. Physicians have noted that contact lens wearers are more likely to develop sensitivity to preservatives in contact lens care solutions, similar to dry-eye patients. All these findings are anecdotal but at least suggest similarities between the dry-eye patient and the contact lens wearer.

The important research finding in dry-eye patients and contact lens wearers supporting the contention that contact lens wear produces tear film disturbance and a dry eye has been the detection of elevated tear osmolarity in contact lens wearers [24]. Phakic daily-wear hard contact lens wearers and phakic extended-wear soft contact lens wearers were found to have significantly elevated mean tear osmolarities compared with those of age- and sex-matched controls ($p < 0.03$ and $p < 0.02$, respectively).

A review of the mechanisms responsible for dry eye reveals that both hard and soft contact lenses have approximately equal potential for producing dry eye [1]. As a result of decreased tearing during sleep, extended wear of soft contact lenses is likely to produce greater ocular surface changes than the daily wearing of soft lenses. Therefore, wearers of extended-wear contact lenses regularly need to instill a saline irrigating solution or artificial tears on awakening in the morning. The degree of deposit formation on contact lenses appears to parallel signs of tear dysfunction commonly associated with dry eye. Infrequent blinking, blepharitis, and entrapment of debris beneath the contact lens indicate ocular surface shedding and inadequate flushing beneath the lens. Lens fit, lens type, and the schedule of lens wear are important factors not only in meeting the cornea's need for oxygen but also in maintaining adequate tear function.

Is Contact Lens Wear Therapeutic for the Dry Eye?

Although it is possible that contact lens wear can serve as a therapeutic measure for the dry eye, I believe the therapeutic effect would be minimal. The presence of a contact lens can stimulate the production of reflex tears, which have been shown to have a higher concentration of the antibacterial enzyme lysozyme, even in the dry-eye patient [1]. A specific type of contact lens has been reported to provide a barrier to evaporation in the dry eye [25], but no convincing data have yet appeared. In most cases, the dry-eye patient is so conscious of eye irritation that the idea of placing any object in the eye to produce relief—even a thin, soft contact lens—is unacceptable. Similarly, I have found that very few dry-eye patients obtain relief from artificial tear inserts that dissolve slowly to bolster the evaporative barrier of the tear film surface [26]. Only to the extent that recurrent erosion may be related to a localized area of drying and an abnormality of the tear base, therapeutic soft contact lenses may be helpful in relieving symptoms and promoting resolution of a possible dry-eye condition [27].

Is Dry Eye a Contraindication to Contact Lens Wear?

Some consider a diagnosis of dry eye an absolute contraindication to contact lens wear. The philosophical stance is similar to an older one that advises against contact lens wear in general because of potential harm to the eye. Clearly, a patient in whom dry eye has been diagnosed who wishes to wear contact lenses accepts a greater risk than the contact lens wearer without a dry-eye condition. The degree of increased risk depends on the severity of the dry eye and patient compliance to prescribed contact lens–wearing schedules and dry-eye therapy.

The severity of the dry-eye condition has been found to vary considerably from individual to individual [28]. In addition, recent studies suggest that tear film abnormalities associated with a dry eye are commonly observed in contact lens wearers [1]. What remains uncertain is whether contact lens wear worsens the dry-eye condition. This question must be answered for each patient individually according to his or her ocular response to contact lens wear.

■ References

1. Farris RL. The dry eye: its mechanisms and therapy with evidence that contact lens wear is a cause. CLAO J 1986;12:234–246
2. Mathers WD, Shields WJ, Sachdev MS, et al. Meibomian gland dysfunction in chronic blepharitis. Cornea 1991;10:277–285
3. Farris RL. Staged therapy for the dry eye. CLAO J 1991;17:207–215
4. Allansmith MR, Ross RN, Greiner JV. Giant papillary conjunctivitis: diagnosis and treatment. In: Dabezies OH, ed. Contact lenses: CLAO guide to basic science and clinical practice. Boston: Little, Brown, 1989:43.1–43.17
5. Hart DE. Contact lens/tear film interactions: depositions and coatings. In: Dabezies OH, ed. Contact lenses, update 7: CLAO guide to basic science and clinical practice. Boston: Little, Brown, 1990:45.A-1–27
6. Boswall GJ, Ehlers WH, Liustro A, Donshik PC. A comparison of conventional and disposable extended wear contact lenses. CLAO J 1993;19:158–165
7. Lemp MA. Surfacing the precorneal tear film. Ann Ophthalmol 1973;22:165–176
8. Mishima S. Pharmacology of ophthalmic solution. Contact Intraocul Lens Med J 1978;4:23–46
9. Mishima S, Gasset A, Klyce SD, Baum JL. Determination of tear volume and tear flow. Invest Ophthalmol 1966;5:264–276
10. Mishima S. Corneal physiology under contact lenses. In: Gasset AR, ed. Soft contact lenses. St Louis: Mosby, 1972:19–36
11. Lemp MA, Holly FJ, Iwata S, Dohlman CH. The precorneal tear film: I. Factors in spreading and maintaining a continuous tear film over the corneal surface. Arch Ophthalmol 1970;83:89–94
12. Norm MS. Mucous thread in inferior conjunctival fornix. Acta Ophthalmol (Copenh) 1966;44:33–42
13. Adams AD. The morphology of human mucus. Arch Ophthalmol 1979;97:730–734
14. Friend J, Kiorpes T, Thoft RA. Conjunctival goblet cell frequency after alkali injury is not accurately reflected by aqueous tear mucin content. Invest Ophthalmol Vis Sci 1983;24:612–618
15. Holly FJ. Tear film physiology and contact lens wear: I. Pertinent aspects of tear film physiology. Am J Optom Physiol Opt 1981;58:324–330
16. Holly FJ. Tear film physiology and contact lens wear: II. Contact lens–tear interaction. Am J Optom Physiol Opt 1981;58:331–341
17. Polack FM, McNiece MT. The treatment of dry eyes with Na hyaluronate (Healon). Cornea 1982;1:133–136
18. Lemp MA, Hamill JR. Factors affecting tear film breakup in normal eyes. Arch Ophthalmol 1973;89:103–105

19. Vanley GT, Leopold IH, Gregg TH. Interpretation of tear film breakup. Arch Ophthalmol 1977;95:445–448
20. Musco PS, Aquavella JV. Therapeutic contact lenses. In: Dabezies OH, ed. Contact lenses: CLAO guide to basic science and clinical practice. Boston: Little, Brown, 1989;46:1–46.16
21. Gilbard JP, Carter JB, Sang DN, et al. Morphologic effect of hyperosmolarity on rabbit corneal epithelium. Ophthalmology 1984;91:1205–1212
22. Holly FJ, Lemp MA. The preocular tear film and dry eye syndromes. Boston: Little, Brown, 1973
23. Thoft RA, Friend J. The ocular surface. Boston: Little, Brown, 1979
24. Farris RL. Tear analysis in contact lens wearers. CLAO J 1986;12:106–111
25. Baldone JA, Kaufman HE. Soft contact lenses and clinical diseases. Am J Ophthalmol 1983;95:851–952
26. Mishima S, Maurice DM. The oily layer of the tear film and evaporation from the corneal surface. Exp Eye Res 1961;1:39–45
27. Kaufman HE. Therapeutic use of soft contact lenses. In: Dabezies OH, ed. Contact lenses: CLAO guide to basic science and clinical practice. Orlando, FL: Grune & Stratton, 1984:46.1–46.11
28. Farris RL. Tear osmolarity variation in keratoconjunctivitis sicca. Trans Am Ophthalmol Soc 1986;84:250–268

Possible Mechanisms of Cellular Activation and Tissue Destruction in Sjögren's Syndrome

Ichiro Saito, D.D.S., Ph.D.

Sjögren's syndrome (SS) is a chronic inflammatory disease of unknown origin, marked by inflammation and destruction of the lacrimal glands and salivary glands. Although the etiology of SS remains elusive, data regarding the pathogenesis of tissue destruction and the mechanisms of cellular activation in the disease continue to accrue at a rapid rate. As in previous years, many recent studies implicate cytokine networks and cell adhesion molecules in perpetuating inflammation of the lacrimal and salivary glands. In addition, studies on granzyme A and perforin expression, as well as intriguing evidence supporting a potential role for infectious agents, also offer novel views of inflammation of these glands. In this chapter, I will review recent advances in these three areas of research.

■ Expression of Cytokines and Cell Adhesion Molecules in SS

Dryness of the mouth and eyes is a characteristic of SS, a chronic autoimmune disease. Impairment of salivary and lacrimal gland function is caused by destruction of acini or ductal cells accompanied by lymphocytic infiltration, which is believed to be immunologically mediated [1]. $CD4^+$ and $CD45RO^+$ T cells are the major subsets infiltrated into the exocrine glands of SS, and B cells frequently appear in the lesion. However, the mechanism for the recruitment of specific lymphocyte subsets in the lesion have not yet been clarified in SS.

Leukocyte adhesion is a crucial step in the development of both normal immune responses and inflammatory processes. Recently, novel cell adhesion molecules, including vascular cell adhesion molecule-1 (VCAM-1), intercellular adhesion molecule-1 (ICAM-1), and E-selectin (endothelial-leukocyte adhesion molecule-1 [ELAM-1]), have been identified [2]. These molecules mediate a variety of cell-cell interactions by binding to leukocyte

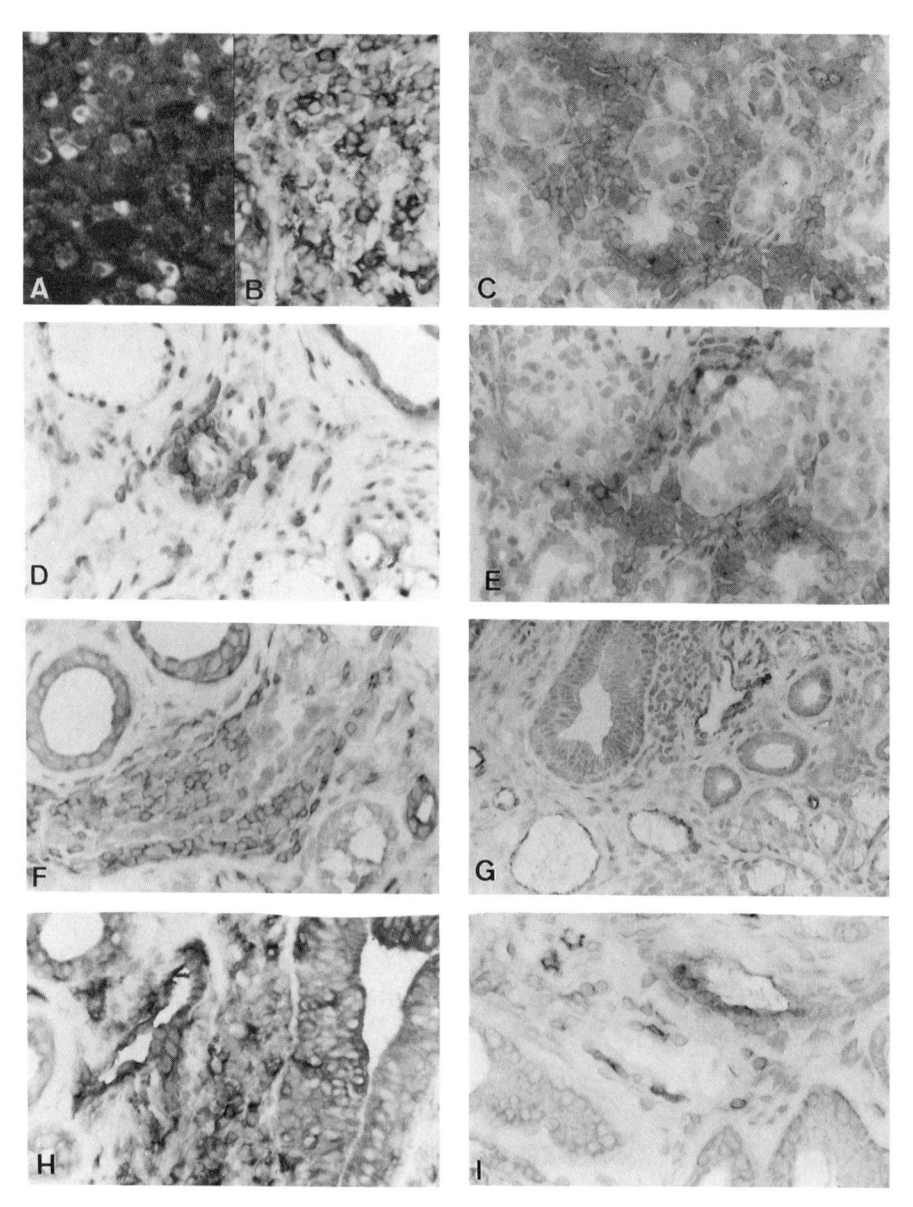

Figure 1 *Immunohistological analysis of Sjögren's syndrome (SS) biopsies. Monoclonal antibodies were used to analyze frozen tissue sections of SS biopsies after acetone fixation. (A) Immunofluorescence staining of salivary gland (SG) of SS for very late antigen (VLA-α4⁺). (B) Immunoperoxidase staining of SG of SS β1 integrin. In the SS lacrimal gland biopsy, clusters of VLA-α4⁺ cells were located near glandular acini (C) and endothelium (D). (E) The distribution of CD45RO on SS SG biopsy was similar to that of VLA-4, and extensive coexpression (>50%) was observed. (F) Tissue sections of the SG of SS were stained with HLA-DR, which reacts with epithelial and lymphocytic cells. (G) Intercellular adhesion molecule-1 (ICAM-1) was faintly expressed by ductal epithelial cells and postcapillary venules. (H) Numerous VCAM-1 positive vessels and some lymphocytic cells were observed in SG of SS. (I) Only rare vessels and lymphocytic cells expressed endothelial-leukocyte adhesion molecule-1 (ELAM-1). (Original magnification in A through F, H, and I, × 400; original magnification in G, × 250.)*

adhesion receptor molecules. They are constitutively expressed in a few cell types but also are induced in a variety of cells in response to inflammatory stimuli in vivo and to cytokines, such as interferon gamma (IFN-γ), tumor necrosis factor (TNF), and interleukin-1 (IL-1) in vitro, suggesting that these molecules are important for regulating immune responses [3–5].

Our study revealed that several features distinguish VCAM-1 and ICAM-1 expression from ELAM-1 at sites of inflammation in SS. Localization of VCAM-1– and ICAM-1–positive cells in salivary and lacrimal gland tissue biopsies appeared to be more limited than those of E-selectin–positive cells. VCAM-1 was detected in postcapillary venules and some mononuclear cells, whereas ICAM-1 was found in epithelial cells (acini or ductal structures), fibroblastic cells, and a few mononuclear cells in salivary glands [6] and lacrimal glands of SS. These observations indicate that overexpression of VCAM-1 and ICAM-1 may simply reflect activation by inflammatory cytokines at sites of immune reactions, since the expression of these cell adhesion molecules occurs concurrently with IFN-γ, and IL-1β expression in salivary and lacrimal glands of SS (Figs 1, 2).

A very recent study by Yednock and colleagues [7] demonstrated that the induction of experimental autoimmune encephalomyelitis (EAE) is prevented by antibodies against very late antigen (VLA-4). They also showed that in vitro binding of lymphocytes and monocytes to inflamed EAE brain vessels was effectively inhibited by anti-VLA-4 antibodies. These data further emphasize the importance of the VLA-4/VCAM-1 pathway in the induction and perpetuation of autoimmune processes in specific organs. Manipulation of the cell adhesion molecule pathways might become a new mode of treatment for certain autoimmune diseases, such as SS.

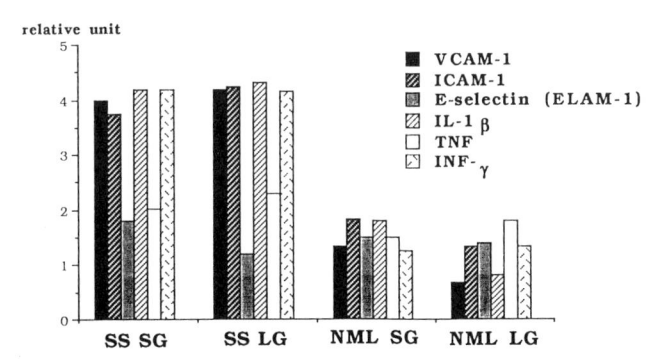

Figure 2 *Semiquantitative analysis of intensity of amplified products by reverse transcriptase polymerase chain reaction of salivary (SG) and lacrimal gland (LG) specimens from Sjögren's syndrome (SS) patients and normal healthy controls (NML). (VCAM-1 = vascular cell adhesion molecule-1; ICAM-1 = intercellular adhesion molecule-1; ELAM-1 = endothelial-leukocyte adhesion molecule-1; IL-1β = interleukin-1 beta; TNF = tumor necrosis factor; INF-γ = interferon gamma.)*

■ Potential Role of Environmental Factors in SS

Studies of autoimmune disease in identical twins have shown a greatly increased concordance rate (i.e., if one twin has the disease, then the second twin has an approximate 20% chance of developing the autoimmune disease). Although this observation indicates the strong role of genetics as a risk factor for pathogenesis, it is important to point out that the majority of twins do not show concordance of disease and also to emphasize the importance of nongenetic factors in pathogenesis. Such nongenetic factors may include exposure to exogenous agents (i.e., environmental antigens) and the occurrence of random recombination events occurring at different genetic loci (i.e., the recombination of immunoglobulin and T-cell antigen receptor variable and constant regions). It is likely that both these factors contribute to the discordance of autoimmune disease among twins and the relatively low proportion of individuals with a specific genotype that actually develops SS.

The environmental cofactor(s) responsible for SS remain unknown. Indirect evidence has supported a role for the Epstein-Barr virus (EBV), because this virus maintains latency in the salivary and lacrimal glands in normals after primary infection. Increased levels of EBV DNA and antibody responses to EBV-encoded proteins have been found in a subset of SS patients in the United States [8], Europe [9], and Japan [10]. Immunohistology and in situ hybridization have suggested that the EBV genome is located in epithelial cells and, to a lesser extent, in B cells [9]. However, the long latent period between initial EBV infection (usually before age 10 years) and the onset of SS (usually after age 25 years) makes it difficult to attribute a primary pathogenic role to EBV. It is possible, however, that EBV becomes reactivated as a consequence of cytokine released in the SS epithelial cell microenvironment and thus is a secondary event (rather than a primary cause) of the autoimmune response. The strong T-cell responses against EBV-encoded antigens in all normals suggest that the reactivation of EBV must be considered a candidate for disease perpetuation, even if it is not the primary cause of disease.

Indirect evidence has also suggested a potential role for retroviruses [11]. In one study, a subpopulation of SS patients had antibodies to human immunodeficiency virus (HIV) retroviral protein p30 [12]. These studies were interpreted to show a role for infection by exogenous retroviruses, analogous to the salivary gland syndrome that occurs in some patients with the acquired immunodeficiency syndrome (AIDS) [13]. However, the significance of these studies remains unclear.

Finally, it is known that in endemic areas of Japan, human T-lymphotropic virus type 1 (HTLV-1) infection may be associated with SS-like symptoms, and the occurrence of a "tax" gene may serve to transactivate important other genes. In a subpopulation of HIV-infected individuals, SS-like conditions may likewise develop [13]. However, the histology and immunohistology of these glandular swellings (i.e., absence of anti-SS and anti-SS B antibodies) and a distinct HLA-DR predisposition (i.e., HLA-DR5) distinguish the HIV-associated condition from primary SS.

■ Control of Lymphoproliferation by Interferon Alpha in SS

Interferon alpha (IFN-α) is a regulatory glycoprotein with distinct biological effects. It is a highly active intercellular mediator that induces viral resistance and inhibits cellular proliferation. IFN-α has two probably related but separate effects on B lymphocytes: It inhibits B-cell proliferation and infection by EBV. Because the complement receptor (C3d) to EBV is also an IFN-α receptor, IFN-α binding to B cells may open new approaches to IFN-α therapy for EBV-related polyclonal B-cell activation, B-cell malignancies, and the possibility of EBV infections [14]. However, the mechanism underlying inhibition of EBV infection and proliferation of EBV-infected B cells by IFN-α is not well established. As for the mechanism of antiproliferative action by IFN-α, previous reports showed that IFN-α can induce a tumor suppressive gene product (RB) whereby the growth of many mammalian cell types, including tumor cells, is inhibited [15].

My colleagues and I [16] have already demonstrated the following as a result of increased excretion of EBV in SS saliva: (1) Levels of EBV DNA in salivary gland biopsies of SS patients are increased. (2) There is spontaneous and massive production of transforming EBV in B-cell lines established from SS patients (SS-BCL). (3) The transfer of SS salivary gland lymphocytes or SS-BCL into severe combined immunodeficiency (SCID) mice reproduced polyclonal B-cell activation and B-cell lymphoma carrying EBV genome similar to those seen in SS. On the basis of these findings, we evaluated the effects of IFN-α in SS.

From our preliminary experiments, IFN-α has an inhibitory effect on EBV-induced transformation of human B lymphocytes by immortalization assay. Moreover, EBV-induced tumorigenesis in SCID mice reconstituted with SS-BCLs is inhibited by IFN-α. Infusion of IFN-α was significantly effective in arresting B-cell tumor growth and induced remission of tumor development. These results suggest that IFN-α may be beneficial for the treatment of the lymphoproliferation seen in SS patients.

■ Granzyme A and Perforin in SS

Tissue destruction of the lacrimal and salivary glands is the cardinal feature of SS. Although lymphocyte infiltration accompanies this destruction, the mechanism of tissue destruction has not been elucidated. Recently, it was suggested that granzyme A and perforin are associated with

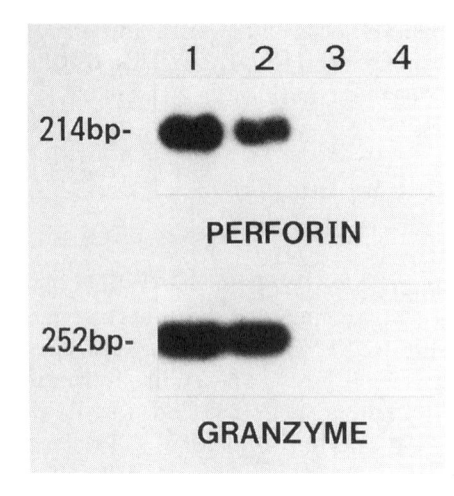

Figure 3 Southern blot analysis of polymerase chain reaction–amplified products of perforin and granzyme A in lacrimal gland biopsies from Sjögren's syndrome patients (lanes 1 and 2), non-Sjögren's syndrome dry-eye patient (lane 3), and normal healthy control (lane 4). All autoradiographs were exposed for 4 hours. The size of the amplification products were 214 base pair (bp) for perforin and 252 bp for granzyme A.

immunologically mediated cytolysis in such autoimmune diseases as rheumatoid arthritis, where the regulation of these compounds in synovial fluid lymphocytes causes tissue destruction [17]. In lacrimal and salivary glands in SS, CD4+ T cells are in direct contact with the glandular cells. Although cytotoxic cells generally are believed to exhibit CD8+ phenotype, activated CD4+ T cells can be induced to exhibit killer function and are recognized by their content of granzyme A and perforin A, two enzymes that mediate the killing process.

Recently, my colleagues and I demonstrated lymphocytes containing granzyme A in SS biopsies (Fig 3) [18], suggesting that activated CD4+ T cells containing this enzyme may destroy epithelial cells expressing a specific antigen on the cell surface presented by class II molecules. The immunosuppressive effects of cyclosporin A on T cells are well-known, which can, in part, be explained by cyclosporine's suppressive action on granzyme A and perforin [19]. Thus, cyclosporin A can be a potent agent for preventing the destruction of the lacrimal and salivary glands in SS through the pathogenic mechanism proposed in this study.

■ References

1. Talal N. Sjögren's syndrome. Curr Opin Immunol 1990;2:622–624
2. Springer TA. Adhesion receptor of the immune system. Nature 1990;346:425–434
3. Pober JS, Gimbone MA Jr, Mendrick DL, et al. Overlapping patterns of activation of human endothelial cells by interleukin 1, tumor necrosis factor, and immune interferon. J Immunol 1986;137:893–896
4. Dustin ML, Springer TA. Lymphocyte function–associated antigen-1 (LFA-1) interaction with intercellular adhesion molecule-1 (ICAM-1) is one of at least three

mechanisms for lymphocyte adhesion to cultured endothelial cells. J Cell Biol 1988; 107:321–331
5. Cotran RS, Pober JS. Endothelial activation: its role in inflammatory and immune reactions. In: Simionescu N, Simionescu M, eds. Endothelial cell biology. New York: Plenum, 1988:335–347
6. St Clair EW, Angellilo JC, Singer KH. Expression of cell-adhesion molecules in the salivary gland microenvironment of Sjögren's syndrome. Arthritis Rheum 1992;35: 62–66
7. Yednock TA, Cannon C, Fritz LC, et al. Prevention of experimental autoimmune encephalomyelitis by antibodies against alpha$_4$ beta$_1$ integrin. Nature 1992;35: 63–66
8. Saito I, Servenius B, Compton T, Fox RI. Detection of Epstein-Barr virus DNA by polymerase chain reaction in blood and tissue biopsies from patients with Sjögren's syndrome. J Exp Med 1989;169:2191
9. Mariette X, Gozlan J, Clerc D, et al. Detection of Epstein-Barr virus DNA by *in situ* hybridization and polymerase chain reaction in salivary glands biopsy specimens from patients with Sjögren's syndrome. Am J Med 1991;90:286
10. Inoue N, Harada S, Miyasaka N, et al. Analysis of antibody titers to Epstein-Barr virus nuclear antigens in sera of patients with Sjögren's syndrome and with rheumatoid arthritis. J Infect Dis 1991;164:22
11. Talal N, Flescher E, Dang H. Evidence of possible retroviral involvement in autoimmune diseases. Ann Allergy 1992;69:22
12. Talal N. Detection of serum antibodies to retroviral proteins in patients with Sjögren's syndrome (autoimmune exocrinopathy). Arthritis Rheum 1990;33:77
13. Itescu S, Brancato LJ, Buxbaum J, et al. A diffuse infiltrative CD8 lymphocytosis syndrome in human immunodeficiency virus (HIV) infection: a host immune response associated with HLA-DR-5. Ann Intern Med 1990;112:3
14. Delcayre AX, Salas F, Mathur S, et al. Epstein-Barr virus/complement C3d receptor is an interferon α receptor. EMBO J 1991;10:919–926
15. Kumar R, Atlas I. Interferon α induces the expression of retinoblastoma gene product in human Burkitt lymphoma Daudi cells: role in growth regulation. Proc Natl Acad Sci USA 1992;89:6599–6603
16. Takeishi M, Saito I, Yamamoto K, Miyasaka N. Spontaneous production of Epstein-Barr virus by B lymphoblastoid cell lines obtained from patients with Sjögren's syndrome. Arthritis Rheum 1993;36:827–835
17. Griffiths G, Alpert S, Lambert E, et al. Perforin and granzyme A expression identifying cytolic lymphocytes in rheumatoid arthritis. Proc Natl Acad Sci USA 1992;89: 549–553
18. Tsubota K, Saito I, Miyasaka N. Expression of perforin and granzyme A in lacrimal glands of patients with Sjögren's syndrome. Am J Ophthalmol, in press
19. Liu C, Rafii S, Granelli-Paperno A, et al. Perforin and serine esterase gene expression in stimulated human T cells. J Exp Med 1989;170:105–118

Punctal Occlusion

David W. Lamberts, M.D.

"The mechanism of the flow of tears into the nasolacrimal duct is not clearly understood, but with the idea in mind that these ducts might be functioning in spite of the diminished amount of secretion, I decided to destroy them and note the effect. In other words, by destroying the conductivity of these ducts, I hoped it would be possible to make better use of the tears that were formed by the atrophied lacrimal glands" [1]. William Beetham wrote these words in 1935 as part of his candidate's thesis for the American Ophthalmology Society. He thus described, for the first time, the procedure of punctal occlusion. Specifically, he advocated electrocautery of the canaliculi. Two years later, MacMillan and Cone [2] also described the closure of the canaliculi by electrocautery in a case of neuroparalytic keratitis.

Since these early descriptions of canalicular occlusion, two opposing criticisms of the technique often have been discussed. One is that the procedure is permanent—that is, it cannot be reversed if problems occur after cautery. The second is that the procedure is not permanent enough—that is, the cauterized canaliculus is prone to reopen in time. Most of the literature about punctal occlusion in the years since its original description has focused on these two problems.

■ Permanent Procedures

Electrocautery

One of the most common techniques to accomplish punctal closure using electrocautery is as follows: Lidocaine hydrochloride 1% (Xylocaine) is used to infiltrate the eyelid adjacent to the punctum and nasally toward the nasolacrimal sac adjacent to the canaliculus. A topical anesthetic is instilled in the cul-de-sac. The electrocautery instrument (Hyfrecator, Birtcher Corp., Los Angeles, CA) is plugged in and the cord inserted into the low-voltage hole. A fine, needle type epilation tip is placed in the handle, and the tip is threaded into the punctum and along the canaliculus for a distance of 10 to 12 mm. With the power setting between number 15 and 20 on the dial, the foot pedal is depressed while the conjunctival side of the canaliculus is observed. A blanching of the conjunctiva signifies cauterization. When this occurs, the tip is pulled 1 to 2 mm out of the canaliculus and the pedal is again depressed. As the tip is withdrawn, the power is continuously decreased. As the tip approaches the punctum, the power should be low (less than 5). Caution must be exercised at this point, because a small amount of power will produce a large amount of burn once the tip is near the eyelid surface.

It should be noted that the power setting varies depending on the instrument. Only one eye should be done at a time, owing to the remote possibility that epiphora will result unexpectedly.

In 1989, Knapp and colleagues [3] studied deep versus superficial punctal occlusion using a two-battery Weck thermal cautery instrument. For the deep method of cauterization, the cautery tip was inserted through the punctum to the full depth of the vertical canaliculus. For the superficial method, the cautery tip was placed against, but not inserted into, the punctum and was turned on. At 1 year, the cumulative risk of a superficial cauterization opening was approximately 60%, whereas that of a deep cauterization was 18% or so.

Even with thorough cauterization, in some patients the canaliculus will reopen in time. Sysi [4], in 1949, described a method of canalicular resection in an effort to prevent this problem. He incised the skin of the eyelid approximately 2 to 3 mm from the edge of the lid and parallel with it. A lacrimal probe was placed in the canaliculus so that it could easily be recognized and isolated. He then cut off the canaliculus just below the punctum and as far nasally as possible. The skin wound was closed with some silk sutures and the punctum destroyed by diathermy. Sysi reported permanent results with this technique.

Laser Cautery

More recently, the argon laser has been used to close the punctum in an effort to obtain permanent occlusion. The technique was originally described by Herrick and modified by Rashad (personal communication, 1986). I perform it in the following fashion: Local anesthetic is used to block the area below the medial canthal ligament just behind the septum and also the infranuclear nerve just above the medial canthal ligament. A violet skin-marking pencil is used to apply pigment to the area around the punctum so that the light from the laser will be absorbed and converted to heat. The power source is used in the continuous mode at 400 mW, and spot size is set at approximately 50 μm. A ring of burns is made around the punctal opening, each nearly 1 mm from the opening, until a full 360 degrees has been cauterized. Then the spot size is increased to 100 μm and the power reduced to 200 mW. The punctum itself, which is now elevated compared to the surrounding depressed burn, is likewise burned. The depth of the crater when finished is approximately 2 to 3 mm. The patient is sent home on no medications.

Recently, Benson and coworkers [5] reported a retrospective study of 20 patients who had undergone laser punctal occlusion. Only 3 of 22 puncta (14%) of laser punctal occlusion patients remained occluded at the time of the authors' examination (13 to 21 months after burning). There was no correlation between status of the punctum and spot size, number of burns, or time to examination. These authors concluded that laser cautery was not effective for long-term punctal occlusion and that thermal or electrodesiccation might be more effective [6].

Glatt [7] has described an interesting case of a 76-year-old woman in whom all four puncta were closed permanently. Eleven weeks after punctal closure, she developed dacryocystitis on the left side. Glatt postulated that the patient probably had preexisting nasolacrimal duct obstruction on that side and that iatrogenic occlusion of the upper and lower puncta created a complete proximate block of the lacrimal outflow tract, which led to the dacryocystitis.

Temporary Procedures

Intracanalicular Gelatin Implants

Because they have been concerned about the permanence of the types of punctal or canalicular occlusion just described, clinicians have devised several ingenious methods of temporarily blocking the outflow channels. Among the first were intracanalicular gelatin implants described by Foulds in 1961 [8]. These were long, slender (0.5-mm × 4-cm) rods of gelatin that were threaded down the canaliculus with forceps. Foulds tried these rods in 9 patients with Sjögren's syndrome or keratoconjunctivitis sicca and reported good results. If there was improvement in the patient's condition, then the canaliculus was closed permanently by cautery after the rods had dissolved.

Cyanoacrylate Tissue Adhesive

In 1976, Patten [9] described the use of N-butyl cyanoacrylate tissue adhesive as a method of temporary punctal closure. The occlusion was performed as follows: One drop of 0.5% proparacaine was used for anesthesia. A cotton-tipped applicator wetted with 4% cocaine was placed on the punctum, and the punctum then was dilated with a punctal dilator. Next a hand-held electric corneal rust remover with a small burr bit was placed in the dilated punctum, and the epithelium was mechanically removed. A sponge was used to dry the punctal area, after which a thin polyethylene tube with a tiny amount of N-butyl cyanoacrylate tissue adhesive stained with methylene blue dye was applied to the crater of the punctum. The lower eyelid was left everted until the tissue adhesive had dried. In 15 treated eyes, the average retention time was 2½ weeks. The glue plug can be removed with jewelers' forceps.

Collagen Implants

Robert Herrick developed small (3-mm-long) collagen implants for canalicular occlusion (Lacrimedics, Inc., Rialto, CA). The implants, made of absorbable collagen, provide temporary (approximately 2 weeks') occlusion of the lacrimal drainage system. They are marketed six to a package and are threaded down into the canaliculus with jewelers' forceps. As a variation on this theme, Girard and associates [10], in 1992, described a method of punctal closure whereby a collagen rod is inserted into the canaliculus and then deep cautery of the punctum and vertical canaliculus is performed. These researchers believe that presence of the collagen plug prevents the passage of tears until cicatrization of the punctum and vertical canaliculus is complete.

Silicone Plugs

Herrick also has developed a canalicular plug (as opposed to the punctal plug). The canalicular plug (Lacrimedics, Inc., Rialto, CA) is shaped like a very skinny funnel but without an opening on the narrow end. This device is impaled on an inserting metal rod, introduced into the punctum, and then pushed all the way down into the canaliculus. In this manner, the silicone does not rest on the punctum and will not touch the eye at any time. If the plug needs to be removed, it can be pushed or irrigated into the nasolacrimal sac.

Perhaps the method of temporary occlusion most commonly used today is the Freeman punctal plug [11]. Originally described in 1975, the plug is now produced by Eagle Vision, Memphis, TN. Technique for inserting the original plug is as follows: First, the eye is anesthetized with a topical anesthetic such as proparacaine hydrochloride or cocaine. The drop should be applied several times and a few minutes should be allowed for maximum anesthesia of the conjunctival surface. Saturated cotton may help achieve this anesthesia. The procedure is done on an outpatient basis and, ideally, with an operating microscope, but a loupe is adequate. Rarely, it may be necessary to anesthetize the eyelids with an injectable agent. The punctum is gently dilated (with the dilator that is enclosed with the plug) to an opening of not more than 1.2 mm, thus protecting the punctal ring from fracture. (In the event of fracture, the punctal ring will heal, but it may never be as tight again.) The punctal plug should have been prepared previously by loading it onto the inserter. While the eyelid is retracted with one hand, the dilator is quickly removed with the other and the plug inserted into the punctum down to the level of the dome head. The punctal ring will rapidly constrict the punctum around the plug. After the plug is placed, the inserter is withdrawn while the plug is held down either with the outside sleeve of the inserter or by pressing down with small forceps on the dome head. If the plug is ineffective, if epiphora results, or if the plug points backward and rubs against the conjunctiva, it can easily be removed with jewelers' forceps.

Partially in response to clinicians' requests, Eagle Vision recently introduced several different-sized plugs to the market. The plugs are now available in smaller sizes (petite, mini, etc.) so that maximum dilation (as described earlier) may no longer be necessary in some patients.

Willis and colleagues [12] studied 18 patients who had aqueous-deficient dry eyes and in whom all four puncta were closed with silicone plugs. Plugs extruded within 2 weeks in 4 of the 18 patients (22%). Three of the 14 patients who retained plugs did not experience any improvement in symptoms. Eleven of 14 (79%) who retained the plugs improved subjectively, and all were able to reduce topical therapy. No patient, however, was able to stop the topical drops completely. Interestingly, the authors report that 3 patients complained of epiphora and each requested that one plug be removed from each eye, but all 3 patients later requested replacement of the plugs!

Since the use of silicone punctal plugs has become popular, it should be no surprise that complications have been described. Rapoza and Ruddat [13] describe 2 patients who developed pyogenic granulomas in response to the presence of silicone punctal plugs. The granulomatous mass resolved after removal of the plugs. Nelson [14] described a case of loss of the silicone plug in the canaliculus from excessive force at insertion and then described a case of scaring (closure) of an inferior punctum 2 weeks after removal of a plug in the lower punctum. Both patients did well. A similar problem with the smaller plugs was described by Maguire and Bartley [15]. Levenson and Hofbaver [16] treated a 29-year-old woman in whom the plug was inadvertently pushed all the way into the canaliculus, requiring an incision through the conjunctiva to retrieve and reposition the plug in its proper place within the punctum. These practitioners also described a 33-year-old man with a similar problem in whom an incision was required to remove a plug embedded in the canaliculus. Considering the huge number of silicone plugs placed, these problems appear rather rare.

Copolymer Punctal Plugs

In 1985, Hamano and colleagues [17] described a new type of punctal plug made of a copolymer of povidone and polymethyl methacrylate. This new plug shrinks to one-third its original volume when dried in air and is rehydrated to its original volume after insertion. The plug is 2 mm long and has three different diameters.

■ References

1. Beetham WP. Filamentary keratitis. Trans Am Ophthalmol Soc 1936;33:413
2. MacMillan JA, Cone W. Prevention and treatment of keratitis neuroparalytica by closure of the lacrimal canaliculi. Arch Ophthalmol 1937;18:352
3. Knapp ME, Frueh BR, Nelson CC, Musch DC. A comparison of two methods of punctal occlusion. Am J Ophthalmol 1989;108:315
4. Sysi R. A suggestion for a new method of closing the lacrimal canals. Acta Ophthalmol (Copenh) 1949;27:409
5. Benson DR, Hemmady PB, Snyder RW. Efficacy of laser punctal occlusion. Ophthalmology 1992;99:618
6. Tuberville AW, Frederick WR, Wood TO. Punctal occlusion in tear deficiency syndromes. Ophthalmology 1982;89:1170
7. Glatt HJ. Acute dacryocystitis after punctal occlusion for keratoconjunctivitis sicca. Am J Ophthalmol 1991;111:769
8. Foulds W. Intra-canalicular gelatin implants in the treatment of kerato-conjunctivitis sicca. Br J Ophthalmol 1961;45:625
9. Patten J. Punctal occlusion with *N*-butyl cyanoacrylate tissue adhesive. Ophthalmic Surg 1976;7:24
10. Girard LJ, Barnett L, Rao R. A simple inexpensive technique for punctal occlusion. Am J Ophthalmol 1992;113:340
11. Freeman JM. Punctal plug; evaluation of a new treatment for dry eyes. Trans Am Acad Ophthalmol 1975;79:874
12. Willis RM, Folberg R, Krachmer JH, Holland EJ. The treatment of aqueous-deficient dry eye with removable punctal plugs. Ophthalmology 1987;94:514
13. Rapoza PA, Ruddat MS. Pyogenic granuloma as a complication of silicone punctal plugs. Am J Ophthalmol 1992;113:454
14. Nelson CC. Complications of Freeman plugs. Arch Ophthalmol 1991;109:923
15. Maguire LJ, Bartley GB. Complications associated with the new smaller size Freeman punctal plug. Arch Ophthalmol 1989;107:961
16. Levenson JE, Hofbaver J. Problems with punctal plugs. Arch Ophthalmol 1989;107:493
17. Homano T, Ohashi Y, Cho Y, et al. A new punctum plug. Am J Ophthalmol 1985;100:619

Abstracts of the Inaugural Meeting of the Pacific Ophthalmic Forum

The inaugural meeting of the Pacific Ophthalmic Forum took place July 25–28, 1992, at the Westin Kauai Lagoons Hotel on the island of Kauai, Hawaii. The meeting was designed to bring together ophthalmologists from the Pacific Basin countries to develop friendships and to share their research and clinical experiences. It was attended by 86 ophthalmologists, 46 from Japan and 40 from the United States. The meeting was very casual, to take full advantage of the informal environs of the island and the pleasant warm weather.

Saturday, July 25, was devoted to the topic of structure, function, dystrophies, and immunology. The topics on Sunday, July 26, were systemic disease, infection, and therapeutics. Monday, July 27, was devoted to ocular surface disease and wound healing, and on Tuesday, July 28, the focus was surgery and complications.

■ Structure, Function, Dystrophies, and Immunology

Palisades of Vogt: Their Clinical Significance
Shigeru Kinoshita   Department of Ophthalmology, Kyoto Prefectural University of Medicine, Kyoto, Japan

The palisades of Vogt (POV), the radial infoldings at the limbocorneal junction, are composed of corneal epithelial stem cells (limbal epithelium) and the epithelium's underlying fibrous tissue. Disappearance of POV accompanied by conjunctival epithelial invasion of the cornea is observed in ocular surface disorders such as chemical injuries, Stevens-Johnson syndrome, ocular pemphigoid, radiation keratitis, aniridia, Salzmann's degeneration, and the like, but not in usual corneal epithelial disorders. These findings indicate that ocular surface disorders can be divided into two major categories on the basis of POV observation and that complete POV disappearance implies limbal epithelial depletion. Moreover, POV tend to become obscure even in normal subjects older than 70 years. A plausible hypothesis is that the stem cells of the corneal epithelium decrease as the age of the subject increases.

Surgical Management of Peripheral Ulcerative Keratitis
Shigeru Kinoshita   Department of Ophthalmology, Kyoto Prefectural University of Medicine, Kyoto, Japan

Keratoepithelioplasty is a surgical procedure that generates corneal epithelial cells from donor lenticles, a kind of corneal epithelial transplantation, originally being aimed at ocular surface reconstruction in chemical injury and other incurable epithelial conditions.

We found this procedure to be far more effective than any other surgical treatment (e.g., conjunctival excision, lamellar keratoplasty, mucosal grafts) in reconstructing the devastated ocular surface in peripheral ulcerative keratitis (*Ophthalmology* 1991). One support for its effectiveness is that fresh donor lenticles placed on the sclera did prevent both invasion of conjunctival tissue and superficial neovascularization. This blockade is attributable primarily to the biological placement of corneal epithelium with superficial corneal stroma, including Bowman's membrane, which prevents the accumulation of immune effector cells and activated fibroblasts in the primary target area (i.e., the ulcerated cornea). Therefore, we believe that keratoepithelioplasty is the operation of choice for peripheral ulcerative keratitis.

Prevalence of Keratoconus in Japan
Chihiro Kobayashi* and Atsushi Kanai† **Department of Ophthalmology, Yatsu Hoken Hospital, and †Department of Ophthalmology, Juntendo University School of Medicine, Tokyo, Japan*

The prevalence of keratoconus in Japan was surveyed by questionnaires in selected university hospitals and an outpatient clinic. At Juntendo University Hospital between January 1962 and December 1984, 1,749 patients with keratoconus were surveyed, of whom 1,214 were male and 435 were female. In 1982 and 1983 at 76 other university hospitals and 1 outpatient clinic, 1,929 patients with keratoconus were surveyed, of whom 1,342 were male and 879 were female. Among them, we used only those in the study who were born between 1954 and 1958, reasoning that these patients had already passed the onset age of keratoconus. Therefore, the prevalence of keratoconus patients in Japan was calculated as 15.4×10^5 for men and 5.7×10^{-8} for women. The estimated number of keratoconus patients in Japan currently is 9,586 (6,888 male and 2,698 female patients). Patients who underwent penetrating keratoplasty comprised 16.7 percent of the total.

Keratitis, Ichthyosis, and Deafness (KID) Syndrome: A Report of 2 Cases
Kaori Araki,* Akira Kiritoshi,* Kohji Nishida,* Yuichi Ohashi,* Keizo Takahashi,* and Shigeru Kinoshita† **Department of Ophthalmology, Osaka University Medical School, Osaka, and †Department of Ophthalmology, Kyoto Prefectural University of Medicine, Kyoto, Japan*

Keratitis, ichthyosis, and deafness, or KID syndrome, designated by Skinner and colleagues in 1981, is considered one phenotype of ectodermal dysplasia. Herein we report 2 Japanese patients exhibiting symptoms consistent with the previous reports in the literature.

Two patients, a 34-year-old man and a 34-year-old woman, displayed hyperkeratosis and papillomatosis of the skin, neurosensory deafness, and bilateral vascularizing keratitis. The epithelial cells in the lower half of the cornea were keratinized to varying degrees, small, and morphologically similar to conjunctival epithelial cells. Bulbar conjunctiva was markedly hyperemic, and perilimbal neovascularization was noted all around the peripheral cornea. The palisades of Vogt were preserved in both cases. These findings suggest that corneal epithelial cells in KID syndrome might undergo abnormal differentiation.

Histamine and Tryptase Levels in Conjunctiva
Kazumi Fukagawa,* Hirohisa Saito,† Noriyuki Azuma,‡ Kazuo Tsubota,§ Yuji Iikura,† and Yoshihisa Oguchi* **Department of Ophthalmology, Keio University, Tokyo; †Department of Allergy and Immunology, National Children's Medical Research Center, Tokyo; ‡Department of Ophthalmology, National Children's Hospital, Tokyo; and §Department of Ophthalmology, Tokyo Dental College, Chiba, Japan*

Using brush cytology to obtain specimens, we measured histamine and tryptase levels in tear and conjunctival epithelial cell suspension of children with allergic conjunctivitis (AC) and vernal keratoconjunctivitis (VKC), and we evaluated the correlation with clinical observations. By slit-lamp examination, we scored conjunctival papillary proliferation, superficial punctate keratopathy, blepharitis, and tear breakup time. Normal volunteers were tested in this same manner. The histamine and tryptase levels in tear samples were below the sensitivities of the measurement. Histamine levels in conjunctival cell suspension were 1.31 ± 1.67 ng/ml in AC, 4.84 ± 6.59 ng/ml in VKC, and 0.02 ± 0.016 ng/ml in controls. Tryptase levels were 33.25 ± 21.03 ng/ml in AC, 28.13 ± 21.84 ng/ml in VKC, and 2.57 ± 0.91 ng/ml in controls. Both the histamine and tryptase levels in AC and VKC were significantly higher than in controls ($p \leq 0.05$), but no significant difference was found between AC and VKC. The histamine-tryptase ratio (H/T) was 0.03 ± 0.03 in AC, 0.16 ± 0.096 in VKC, and 0.01 ± 0.01 in controls. We recognized a very high H/T ratio (0.26 ± 0.06) in 2 cases of VKC with severe keratitis. We found the histamine-tryptase ratio correlates with superficial punctate keratitis ($r^2 = 0.72$) and tear breakup time ($r^2 = 0.56$) but not with other clinical findings. From these data, we concluded that the histamine-tryptase levels in conjunctival epithelium obtained by brush cytology is a useful, objective tool to evaluate ocular surface conditions in patients with AC and VKC.

Platelet-Activating Factor in Ocular Inflammatory and Immunological Disorders: Current Knowledge and Potential Investigations
Kevin W. Croft Division of Ophthalmology, Texas A&M University, College of Medicine, and Scott & White Memorial Hospital and Clinic, Temple, Texas

Platelet-activating factor (PAF) is a potent phospholipid mediator of inflammation, and recent evidence implicates its role in the immune response. The historical name given to this compound may lead one to conclude that it influences only its original cell of discovery, when in fact PAF has been shown to be synthesized by and, in turn, influence a multitude of cells including neutrophils, monocytes, endothelial cells, and lymphocytes. Synthetic, nontoxic PAF antagonists have been developed to investigate this mediator's contribution to physiological and pathophysiological processes.

Corticosteroids have remained the mainstay of treatment for numerous ocular disorders, despite significant potential side effects. Considering the potential side effects and relatively nonspecific antiinflammatory and immunosuppressive effects of corticosteroids, their ubiquitous presence in the ophthalmologist's therapeutic armamentarium indicates a need to study the antiinflammatory and immunomodulatory effects of alternative nontoxic agents such as PAF antagonists.

Spheroidal Keratopathy Associated with Subepithelial Corneal Amyloidosis
Ruth M. Santo,,† *Tatsuo Yamaguchi,*,‡ *and Atsushi Kanai** *Department of Ophthalmology, and †Department of Pathology, Juntendo University, and ‡Department of Ophthalmology, St. Luke's International Hospital, Tokyo, Japan

The authors studied, clinically and histopathologically, a peculiar case of primary spheroidal degeneration associated with subepithelial corneal amyloidosis. The spheroidal deposits were observed in the basement membrane, Bowman's layer, and anterior stroma, whereas the amyloid was found in the subepithelial region. The droplets showed characteristic autofluorescence and positive staining with Verhoff's iron hematoxylin. The immunohistochemical study of the amyloid showed negative staining with antibodies to amyloid proteins AA, AP, and light chains (kappa and lambda). This study excluded the possibility of gelatinous droplike corneal dystrophy, which showed positive staining with antibody against the AP component in the same study. To the best of our knowledge, this is the first description of primary spheroidal keratopathy associated with secondary subepithelial corneal amyloidosis in a case that was not subjected to previous operations.

Cytokines and Cell Adhesion Molecules in the Human Cornea
Yoshitsugu Tagawa, Fumihiko Kitagawa, and Hidehiko Matsuda Department of Ophthalmology, Hokkaido University School of Medicine, Sapporo, Japan

We examined 5 corneal buttons obtained at keratoplasty from patients with herpetic stromal keratitis and 2 from patients with keratoconus to clarify by immunohistochemical methods the expression of cytokines, cell adhesion molecules, and immunological receptors in the human cornea. The following monoclonal antibodies were used: anti-IL-1, IL-6, TNF, GM-CGF, ICAM-1, ELAM-1, VCAM-1, CDw29, CD44, and Fc receptor for IgG.

The epithelium of all corneas stained positively for IL-1, IL-6, TNF, CDw29, CD44, and Fc receptor. In the stroma, keratocytes in herpetic stromal keratitis were positive for IL-1, IL-6, ICAM-1, and CD44, whereas keratocytes in keratoconus expressed only CD44. The endothelium of the examined corneas showed positivity for ICAM-1, CDw29, and Fc receptor.

These findings indicate that the human cornea expresses many kinds of cytokines, cell adhesion molecules, and immunological receptors in either inflammatory conditions or its normal state.

Lattice Corneal Dystrophy Types I and III: Clinical, Histological, and Electron-Microscopical Differences

Tetsuo Hida Department of Ophthalmology, Kyorin University School of Medicine, Japan

Lattice corneal dystrophy type III is a newly recognized clinical entity. It has clinical features different from classical type I lattice dystrophy, including very late onset, no episodes of recurrent epithelial erosions, much thicker lattice lines, and mostly sporadic occurrence. Numerous amyloid deposits, some of which are extremely large, are scattered throughout the corneal stroma, located predominantly midway between the epithelium and the endothelium. The epithelial and Bowman's layers generally retain their normal structures.

Morphological and Histochemical Studies of the Development of Human Conjunctival Goblet Cells

Tetsuo Hida,* Kimio Miyashita,† and Noriyuki Azuma‡ *Department of Ophthalmology, Kyorin University School of Medicine; †Department of Ophthalmology, Tokai University School of Medicine; and ‡National Children's Hospital, Tokyo, Japan

Morphological and histochemical characteristics of the human conjunctival goblet cells at the developmental stages were studied using 56 eyes of human embryos and fetuses ranging in age from 5 to 41 weeks of gestation. Goblet cells, which extended to the palpebral and bulbar conjunctiva, appeared in the forniceal area at 8 weeks. Alcian blue staining and the enzyme digestion method revealed the existence of sialic acid in these cells from 9 weeks. We concluded that goblet cells begin to develop from the forniceal area, and they have the same histochemical characteristics in the very early stage as those in the adult, containing mainly sialic acid as glycosaminoglycans.

Scanning and Transmission Electron-Microscopical Studies of the Developing Human Corneal Endothelium

Tetsuo Hida,* Hiroshi Ijichi,* Minoru Fukuda,† and Noriyuki Azuma‡ *Department of Ophthalmology and †Laboratory for Electron Microscopy, Kyorin University School of Medicine, and ‡National Children's Hospital, Tokyo, Japan

The ultramicrostructure of the human corneal endothelium was examined by scanning and transmission electron microscopy. The samples were of 26 human eyes taken from fetuses ranging in age from 5 to 22 weeks of gestation and from a 10-month-old newborn. Corneal endothelium appeared at the seventh or eighth week of gestation, initially forming an irregular structure of two to three layers. From 17 weeks, the corneal endothelial cells composed a single layer and had assumed the form of cuboidal epithelium. These cells showed numerous microvilli protruding toward the anterior chamber. The microvilli disappeared by the twentieth week and, subsequently, a single narrow cilium appeared in the center of each cell. Each cilium had an axial filament complex structure. The cilia involuted with development and were barely visible by 10 months after birth.

■ Systemic Disease, Infection, and Therapeutics

CT-112 and Diabetic Keratopathy
Yuichi Ohashi,* Hisashi Hosotani,* Mamoru Matsuda,* Masakatsu Fukuda,* Kazuo Tsubota,† and Masakazu Yamada‡   *Department of Ophthalmology, Osaka University Medical School, Osaka; †Department of Ophthalmology, Tokyo Dental College, Chiba, and ‡Department of Ophthalmology, Keio University School of Medicine, Tokyo, Japan

The diabetic cornea is latently abnormal and at risk of developing a variety of anomalies after undue stresses such as intraocular operation. For example, diabetic patients often display decreased corneal sensitivity or varying degrees of pleomorphism or polymegarythm in corneal epithelium and endothelium. Abnormal activation of aldose reductase, a key enzyme in the polyol pathway, has been implicated as a pathogenetic mechanism in diabetes mellitus–related complications. Consequently, the clinical efficacy of aldose reductase inhibitors (ARIs) has been extensively explored in recent years.

When topically applied, CT-112, an ARI, has been shown to improve corneal sensitivity and partially to normalize abnormal corneal cell morphology as early as 1 month after treatment initiation. In addition, recurrent corneal erosion and prolonged punctate epithelial keratopathy have been successfully treated with topical CT-112. Topical CT-112 may be useful in treating or preventing corneal complications in diabetic patients.

Pathogenesis of Idiopathic Corneal Endotheliitis
Yuichi Ohashi, Shigeru Kinoshita, Kohji Nishida, and Shuji Yamamoto   Department of Ophthalmology, Osaka University Medical School, Osaka, Japan

Idiopathic corneal endotheliitis, first reported by Khodadoust and Attazadeh in 1982, is characterized by peripherally shifted, progressively advancing corneal stromal edema and a group of keratic precipitates localized along the margin of the edema. There occurs a profound corneal endothelial cell loss, often leading to irreversible bullous keratopathy. Herpes simplex virus DNAs have been repeatedly demonstrated in the aqueous humor of 1 patient with active disease. In our experience, idiopathic corneal endotheliitis predominantly affects adult men, essentially runs a progressive course with frequent recurrence, and responds well to systemic or topical acyclovir.

Timolol-in-GELRITE: A New Vehicle to Enhance Efficacy
Norman S. Levy and Cynthia Alsbury   Florida Ophthalmic Institute, Gainesville, Florida

Timolol is a well-established, nonspecific adrenergic beta-blocker for the treatment of glaucoma. It is usually applied every 12 hours. Reducing the frequency of application to once daily for intraocular pressure control requires enhancing the duration of efficacy. This was achieved using a vehicle that changed from a solution to a gel under the proper ionic conditions, such that the residence time of the drug on the epithelial surface of the cornea and the time for absorption into the anterior chamber were extended. The concentration of GELRITE in the ophthalmic preparation permits the solution to be delivered through the tip of an OCUMETER; it then forms a gel on the corneal surface after contact with the precorneal tear fluid.

Twenty-one patients with an intraocular pressure of at least 23 mm Hg in one or both eyes who were off antiglaucoma medications were enrolled in this study. Each patient was randomly assigned to receive either 0.5% timolol every 12 hours in both eyes or 0.5% timolol-in-GELRITE every 24 hours in both eyes. The patients and physicians were masked to the medication being used. Based on the analysis of our subset of data from a larger multicentered study, timolol-in-GELRITE is well-tolerated and effective for intraocular pressure reduction with a single daily instillation in the morning. The duration of maximal effect exceeds 24 hours when the drug is instilled once daily for a period of more than 2 weeks. The effect is comparable to that achieved with timolol alone when instilled twice daily.

Kinetic Study of Major Histocompatibility Antigen Expression and Lymphocyte Infiltration in Murine Herpetic Keratitis

Toshihiko Uno,* Kozaburo Hayashi,† and Yuichi Ohashi*   **Osaka University Medical School, Osaka, and †Public Health Research Institute of Kobe City, Kobe, Japan*

Herpes simplex virus type 1 (HSV-1) antigen expression, class I and II major histocompatibility (MHC) antigen induction, and $L3T4^+$ or $Lyt2^+$ cell infiltration were analyzed immunohistochemically during the acute phase of murine herpetic keratitis. HSV-1 antigens were detectable in the corneal epithelium at 2 days postinfection and then extended to the superficial stroma at 5 days postinfection. Class I MHC antigens ($H-2^d$) were expressed in all layers of infected as well as uninfected corneas. Class II MHC antigens (Ia^d) were undetectable in uninfected corneas, but they were found in the superficial stroma 2 days postinfection and then spread through the entire stroma. $L3T4^+$ (helper-inducer) cells infiltrated the peripheral stroma at 2 days postinfection, spreading to the central stroma at 5 days postinfection. $Lyt2^+$ (suppressor-cytotoxic) cells also accumulated in the corneal stroma by the fifth postinfection day.

Different Susceptibilities to Corneal Herpes Simplex Virus Type 1 Infection in 2 Inbred Mouse Strains

Shigeki Okamoto,* Kaoru Araki,* Yoshitsugu Inoue,* Yuichi Ohashi,* Kozaburo Hayashi,† and Tetsuo Kase‡   **Department of Ophthalmology, Osaka University Medical School, Osaka; †Public Health Research Institute of Kobe City, Kobe; and ‡Osaka Prefectural Institute of Public Health, Osaka, Japan*

We studied local factors that influence different susceptibilities of corneal herpes simplex virus type 1 (HSV-1) infection in two inbred mouse strains. HSV-1 (CHR-3 strain) was instilled into the conjunctival sac of both DBA/2 and AKR/3 strains. In half the specimens of each strain, the cornea had been scarified. Biomicroscopical examination of corneal lesions was performed every 2 days postinfection. Those mice that had been inoculated with HSV-1 without corneal scarification were sacrificed at 2 days postinfection. Eyeballs, conjunctiva, and eyelids of each strain were excised and homogenized. The virus titers of various organs were estimated.

Dendritic lesions were seen in 94 percent of the DBA/2 mice after HSV-1 inoculation into the conjunctival sacs without corneal scarification. In contrast, none of the AKR/3 mice developed corneal lesions. When corneas of both strains had been scarified before virus inoculation, they developed severe dendritic ulcers at 3 days postinfection.

The extent of virus growth in the conjunctiva and eyelids was compared in both strains. In DBA/2 mice, virus grew better in the conjunctiva, whereas in AKR/3 mice, the eyelids supported better virus growth.

Two Cases of Herpetic Keratitis Caused by an Acyclovir-Resistant Strain

Yoshitsugu Inoue, Yasuko Mori, Yufeng Yao, Satoshi Kawaguchi, Yasutaka Uchihori, and

Yuichi Ohashi Department of Ophthalmology, Osaka University Medical School, Osaka, Japan

Two cases of herpetic keratitis caused by an acyclovir-resistant disease strain are reported. Patient 1, a 37-year-old man with typical dendritic keratitis, was treated by a local ophthalmologist with topical 3% acyclovir ointment two times daily for 2 weeks, with no resolution. In our clinic, the treatment regimen was changed to mechanical debridement of the lesion and topical acyclovir ointment five times daily. However, 2 days later the morbidity of the ulcer remained unchanged. From this point, the patient was given 1% trifluorothymidine every 2 hours and 0.1% idoxuridine every hour. The virus-induced ulcer gradually diminished.

Patient 2, a 34-year-old man, was treated topically as well as systemically with acyclovir and steroids for the diagnosis of stromal herpes virus infection. He eventually developed a typical dendrite, for which mechanical debridement of the lesion and topical acyclovir ointment over 1 week were not effective. When 1% trifluorothymidine eye drops were applied every 2 hours for 3 days, the dendritic ulcer healed completely.

In both cases, herpes simplex virus was isolated from the corneal epithelial lesion. In vitro drug sensitivity testing revealed that both strains were acyclovir-resistant (median effective dose in Patient 1, 8.2 µg/ml; in Patient 2, 3.4 µg/ml).

A Rapid Type Identification of Keratoconjunctivitis-Causing Human Adenoviruses by Restriction Endonuclease Analysis of Polymerase Chain Reaction–Amplified DNA Products

Tetsuo Kase, Akiko Maeda, Yoshiichi Minekawa, Shigeki Okamoto, and Yuichi Ohashi Osaka Prefectural Institute of Public Health and Department of Ophthalmology, Osaka University Medical School, Osaka, Japan

We attempted to diagnose adenoviral keratoconjunctivitis using the polymerase chain reaction (PCR) method coupled with a subsequent restriction endonuclease analysis. Primers for the hexon-coding region were generally useful for all of the adenoviruses investigated (Allard and colleagues, 1990): The amplified DNAs in this system were specifically reactive to keratoconjunctivitis-causing adenoviruses. Amplified, adenovirus-specific DNAs were detectable in the conjunctival swab specimens from which no infectious virus was recovered. Obtained PCR-amplified products, when digested with *RsaI*, *HaeIII*, and *HpaII* enzymes, displayed distinguished electrophoretic profiles depending on each endonuclease used. With this procedure, seven types of keratoconjunctivitis-associated adenoviruses could be clearly identified. For example, several virus isolation–negative conjunctival swab specimens, which had been obtained during the nosocomial type 8 keratoconjunctivitis outbreak in our institution, have demonstrated electrophoretic patterns consistent with type 8 adenovirus. Thus, this restriction endonuclease analysis is a rapid and useful maneuver for typing a keratoconjunctivitis-causing adenoviral agent and is applicable to virus isolation–negative specimens.

Effects of Topical Aldose Reductase Inhibitor (CT-112) on Corneal Sensitivity of Diabetic Rats

Hisashi Hosotani,* Yuichi Ohashi,* Shigeru Kinoshita,* Yasuo Ishii,† Takashi Awata,‡ and Takahiro Matsumoto‡ *Department of Ophthalmology, Osaka University Medical School, Osaka; †Eye Institute of the Cataract Foundation, Tokyo; and ‡Itami Research Laboratories, Senju Pharmaceutical Co., Ltd., Itami, Japan

It is well-known that corneal sensitivity in diabetic patients is decreased. This study was undertaken to investigate whether the topical aldose reductase inhibitor (ARI) CT-112 could reverse the decreased corneal sensitivity in diabetic animals. Streptozocin-induced (70 mg/kg) diabetic rats were divided into two groups, A and B. Group A (n = 15) was treated with 0.25% CT-112 eye drops (four times per day, 5 µl per time), and group B (n = 15) received vehicle eye drops (same frequency and dose) and served as a control. Normal rats (group C, n = 15) were also treated with vehicle eye drops. We measured the corneal sensitivity in each group of rats by Cochet-Bonnet's esthesiometer. The corneal sensitivity in groups A, B, and C after 6 months of treatment was 53 ± 6, 44 ± 4, and 51 ± 4 mm, respectively (mean ± S.D.). There were statistically significant differences between groups A and B ($p = 0.0017$) and between groups B and C ($p = 0.0017$). There was no statistically significant difference between groups A and C. The decreased corneal sensitivity in diabetic rats returned to a normal level after topical ARI treatment.

Clinical and Bacteriological Features of Bacterial Keratitis in the Last 6 Years
Kazuko Kitagawa, Koichi Asano, and Kazuyuki Sasaki   Department of Ophthalmology, Kanazawa Medical University, Uchinada, Japan

Fifty-three cases of bacterial keratitis seen in our clinic from 1985 to 1990 were studied. The major predisposing causative factors were corneal foreign bodies, contact lens use, and corneal scratches. Sixty-seven bacterial strains were detected from 35 cases. Fifty-eight of these strains were gram-positive, and *Staphylococcus epidermidis*, *Corynebacterium* species, and *Staphylococcus aureus* being prominent among them. Only nine strains were gram-negative, and *Moraxella* and *Serratia* organisms were detected in 2 or more cases. Hypopyon developed in 7 cases. The visual outcome in 45 cases was better than 0.2, and no eyes were blinded or lost.

Possible Involvement of Respiratory Syncytial Virus in Allergic Conjunctivitis
Hiroshi Fujishima,* Kazuo Tsubota,* Yoshitaka Okamoto,† and Ichiro Saito‡   *Department of Ophthalmology, Tokyo Dental College, Chiba; †Department of Otolaryngology, Akita University School of Medicine; and ‡Department of Virology and Immunology, Medical Research Institute, Tokyo Medical and Dental University, Tokyo, Japan

Allergic conjunctivitis has been studied for many years, but its pathogenesis remains unknown. Respiratory syncytial virus (RSV) is a unique respiratory pathogen, and its specific immune mechanism has recently been considered to be related to allergic reaction. We investigated the possible involvement of RSV in allergic conjunctivitis.

Using the brush cytology technique, we collected conjunctival epithelium from 30 allergic conjunctivitis patients and 20 controls. For the detection of RSV, we used the RT–polymerase chain reaction (PCR) and confirmed our findings by nested PCR.

RSV sequences were detected in 7 patient samples (23 percent) and in 1 control (5 percent). This result suggested that PCR can detect RSV and that RSV may play an important role in the pathogenesis of allergic conjunctivitis.

Inhibition of Phacoemulsification Probe–Induced Free Radicals by Hyaluronic Acid Viscous Material
Shigeto Shimmura,* Kazuo Tsubota,‡ Yoshihisa Oguchi,* Dai Fukumura,† and Makoto Suematsu†   *Departments of Ophthalmology and †Internal Medicine, Keio University School of Medicine, Tokyo, and ‡Department of Ophthalmology, Tokyo Dental College, Chiba, Japan

We have recently reported the formation of oxygen free radicals by conventional phacoemulsification probes, which may have adverse effects on the corneal endothelium during surgery. In this study, we investigated the effects of commercial hyaluronic acid viscous material (Healon) on such radicals in vitro.

Radical formation was visualized by chemiluminescence and an ultrasensitive photon-counting camera. Results indicated that the viscous material both significantly decreased total luminescence and inhibited the diffusion of radicals originating from the probe tip. This suggests that Healon provides mechanical as well as chemical protection for endothelium against oxidative stress during phacoemulsification.

Ocular Surface Disease and Wound Healing

Observation of the Corneal Epithelium In Vivo
Kazuo Tsubota   Tokyo Dental College and Ichikawa General Hospital, Chiba, Japan

Specular microscopical observation is essential for evaluating the corneal endothelium because it allows cells to be studied without interfering with the cornea. Cell size and shape are important as these characteristics are directly affected by endothelial functions and abnormalities. With the recent development of a special contact lens that provides high-contrast in vivo epithelial pictures, using the specular microscope offers new possibilities for epithelial study. The special contact lens has the same refractive index as the corneal stroma, and this produces a similar relationship between the contact lens and epithelium and the corneal stroma and endothelium. This technique allows the epithelium to be observed in vivo.

Basic Application of Brush Cytology in Conjunctiva
Kazuo Tsubota   Tokyo Dental College and Ichikawa General Hospital, Chiba, Japan

To collect conjunctival cells efficiently, we developed a special brush that is a modification of the Cytobrush used in cervical cytology. The conjunctival brush is small and consists of nylon bristles. Cells collected by such a brush were rinsed into a buffered solution from which filter preparations were made. This technique produced adequate cellular samples from temporal bulbar conjunctiva, and the preparations stained well with the Papanicolaou stain. Under normal conditions, three cell types are observed in the brushing samples: One is the polygonal epithelial cell, the second is the small rounded cell, and the third is a mucus-secreting goblet cell. Irritation caused by the brushing is of the same intensity as irritation caused by collecting cytological specimens by impression or by using cotton swabs.

Dry Eye: New Diagnostic Approaches and Therapy
Kazuo Tsubota   Tokyo Dental College and Ichikawa General Hospital, Chiba, Japan

Dry eye, or keratoconjunctivitis sicca, is caused by abnormalities in the quantity or quality of the tear film layer. Sjögren's syndrome is one typical cause, but other types of dry eye exist. This study presents a classification of three different types of dry eye, differentiated according to their autoimmune status.

A total of 116 dry-eye patients (6 men and 110 women; mean age, 52.2 ± 14.2 years) were enrolled in the study. They were divided into the following three groups: (1) simple dry eye (SDE)—dry eye with no circulating autoantibodies; (2) autoimmune positive dry eye (ADE)—dry eye with circulating autoantibodies; and (3) Sjögren's syndrome (SS)—dry eye associated with Sjögren's syndrome.

Schirmer test results for the three groups were 3.0 ± 2.2 mm in SDE, 3.1 ± 2.0 mm in ADE, and 2.4 ± 2.3 mm in SS, reflecting the inadequacy of this test to differentiate among the groups. However, the results of the Schirmer test with nasal stimulation were 19.1 ± 12.4 mm in SDE and 16.4 ± 10.9 mm in ADE, which were significantly higher than 7.0 ± 6.6 mm in SS ($p < 0.01$). Moreover, rose bengal and fluorescein staining scores were significantly lower in SDE and ADE than in SS. Brush cytology of the conjunctiva revealed more keratinized epithelial cells with inflammatory cells in SS than in either SDE or ADE.

These results showed that SDE and ADE are associated with good reflex tearing and relatively mild alterations of the conjunctiva, whereas in SS there is less reflex tearing and more squamous metaplasia. Although ADE has an autoimmune basis, this type of dry eye should be distinguished from SS.

64Kd Keratin Expression in Normal Conjunctival Epithelium
Akira Kiritoshi,* Kaori Araki,* Koji Nishida,* Yuichi Ohashi,* Tung-Tien Sun,† and Shigeru Kinoshita* *Department of Ophthalmology, Osaka University Medical School, Osaka, Japan, and †Department of Dermatology and Pharmacology, New York University Medical School, New York

Conjunctival epithelium, together with corneal epithelium, comprises the ocular surface. In our clinical experience with conjunctival transplantation, human conjunctival epithelium behaves like corneal epithelium when regenerated on the denuded corneal surface. To better understand the nature of conjunctival epithelial differentiation, we immunohistochemically investigated keratin expression of normal and regenerating rabbit conjunctival epithelium using monoclonal antibody against 64Kd (specific to corneal epithelium, AE5) and other keratins (AE1).

In one study, bulbar and tarsal conjunctival epithelium with eyelid and cornea were excised from normal Japanese albino rabbits. In another study, conjunctival tissues including underlying sclera were excised at 1, 2, 3, 7, and 14 days after a circular conjunctival wound of 7-mm diameter was created by n-heptanol. These samples were immediately cryosectioned and stained for AE5 and AE1. The staining for the 64Kd keratin was intensely observed in the epithelial cells around the fornix and eyelid margin and sparsely in bulbar and tarsal conjunctival epithelium. Regenerating conjunctival epithelium was also shown to express AE5. AE1 was always positive in both normal and regenerating conjunctival epithelium.

These data have revealed that some groups of conjunctival epithelial cells closely resemble corneal epithelial cells, even in a normal state, regarding keratin expression.

Superior Limbic Keratoconjunctivitis and Vitamin A Therapy
Fumihiko Kitagawa, Yoshitsugu Tagawa, and Hidehiko Matsuda Department of Ophthalmology, Hokkaido University School of Medicine, Sapporo, Japan

We examined 10 patients—3 men and 7 women—with superior limbic keratoconjunctivitis. The patients ranged in age from 26 to 60 years. Five patients had thyroid diseases, and 1 had Sjögren's syndrome.

We treated 4 patients with topical vitamin A eye drops and 4 with oral vitamin A. Topical application of vitamin A showed marked decreases of rose bengal staining and hyperemia of the upper bulbar conjunctiva as well as improvement of subjective ocular symptoms, whereas systemic vitamin A failed to improve both clinical findings and subjective symptoms. These findings indicate that vitamin A eye drops are useful for treating superior limbic keratoconjunctivitis.

Effect of Antibiotics on Microbial Contamination of Donor Eyes
Koichi Soya*,† and Mitsuru Sawa‡ *Department of Ophthalmology, University of Tokyo School of Medicine, Tokyo; †Department of Ophthalmology, Asahi General Hospital; and ‡Section of Corneal Transplantation, University Hospital, University of Tokyo School of Medicine, Tokyo, Japan

The effect of changes in antibiotics on the microbial contamination of donor eyes was studied. Donor eyes were enucleated using sterile instruments and were preserved in a whole-eye preservation medium (EP-II supplemented with antibiotics) at 4°C. After corneal buttons were trephined for transplantation, residual corneoscleral tissues were examined. Antibiotics were changed from penicillin G sodium (1,000 units/ml) and colistin sulfate (5,000 units/ml) (group A) to gentamicin sulfate (100 µg/ml) and cefmenoxime hemihydrochloride (1 mg/ml) (group B) in May 1991. Eighty-eight consecutive eyes preserved as group A and 42 eyes as group B were studied. The positive rate of microbial culture was 30.7 percent for group A and 33.3 percent for group B. However, a decrease of *Pseudomonas aeruginosa* and an increase of *Enterobacter* organisms occurred due to the change in antibiotics. In both groups, there were no significant differences in donor age, enucleation time, or preservation time between the positive and negative cases.

Corneal Epithelial Wound Healing in the Denervated Eye
Kaoru Araki,* Yuichi Ohashi,* and Shigeru Kinoshita† *Department of Ophthalmology, Osaka University Medical School, Osaka, and †Department of Ophthalmology, Kyoto Prefectural University of Medicine, Kyoto, Japan

We investigated the effects of surgical trigeminal nerve amputation on corneal epithelial wound healing. A corneal epithelial defect of 10-mm diameter was created in bilateral eyes of 7 New Zealand albino rabbits by n-heptanol. The epithelial healing rate was calculated using photographs taken every 12 hours. The experiment was repeated in the same protocol after the wound was completely closed (14 days later). The average rate of epithelial healing was $1.05 + 0.21$ mm^2 per hour in the denervated cornea and $1.26 + 0.24$ mm^2 per hour in the untreated cornea, a difference that was statistically significant ($p < 0.05$).

In another study, 6 rabbits were mechanically keratectomized. Although the epithelial wound healed completely within 6 days in all control corneas, 5 of 6 rabbits (83 percent) in which the trigeminal nerve had been amputated eventually developed a persistent epithelial defect. Thus, the trigeminal nerve plays an important role in corneal epithelial wound healing.

Dry Eye in Diabetes Mellitus
Yoko Ogawa,* Izumi Kamoshita,* Kenichi Yoshino,† Masafumi Ono,‡ and Kazuo Tsubota§ *Department of Ophthalmology, Tokyo Saiseikai Central Hospital, Tokyo; †Department of Ophthalmology, Yamato City Hospital, Yamato; ‡Department of Ophthalmology, Minami Tama Hospital; and §Department of Ophthalmology, Tokyo Dental College and Ichikawa General Hospital, Chiba, Japan

Sixty eyes of 30 diabetic patients were examined to find the degree of dry eye compared to age- and sex-matched controls. Ninety percent of diabetic patients showed superficial keratoepitheliopathy. In our study, diabetic patients demonstrated significantly reduced tear production and reduced corneal sensation compared to the control group. There was no correlation between tear production and corneal sensation. Nonetheless, in diabetics with dry eye, complaints were relatively rare, probably because these patients have reduced corneal sensation.

Seven Cases of Diabetic Postvitrectomy Keratoepitheliopathy Successfully Treated by Anterior Stromal Puncture
Hisashi Hosotani, Tsunehiko Ikeda, and Yasuo Tano Department of Ophthalmology, Osaka University Medical School, Osaka, Japan

We treated by means of anterior stromal puncture 7 patients with diabetic postvitrectomy keratoepitheliopathy with severe recurrent erosion. We devised a double-barbed, 26-gauge disposable needle for this procedure, which can be performed easily and safely. No previous treatments, such as use of a pressure patch or aldose reductase inhibitor eye drops, had been effective. All 7 patients suffered from adhesion disorders of the corneal epithelium. Each patient was treated successfully by anterior stromal puncture. No recurrences have been seen for 3 to 4 years since treatment. To our knowledge, this is the most effective treatment modality for severe recurrent erosion of various types.

The Effect of Extended-Wear Soft Contact Lenses in Gelatinous Drop–Like Corneal Dystrophy

Kazuhisa Miyamoto,* Yuichi Ohashi,† and Shigeru Kinoshita‡ *Department of Ophthalmology, Nissei Hospital, Osaka; †Department of Ophthalmology, Osaka University Medical School, Osaka; and ‡Department of Ophthalmology, Kyoto Prefectural University of Medicine, Kyoto, Japan

We examined the effect of extended-wear soft contact lenses in 8 patients with gelatinous drop–like corneal dystrophy. This treatment for more than 1 month's duration resulted in decreased subepithelial deposits, reduction of ocular surface inflammation, and improvement of corneal clarity in 5 patients. Additionally, subjective symptoms of these patients (i.e., photophobia, foreign-body sensation, and epiphora) diminished remarkably. In the other 3 patients, extended-wear soft contact lens wear was discontinued because of the ocular pain caused by tight fitting. Environmental changes around the corneal epithelium that are induced by soft contact lens wear may be responsible for this phenomenon.

Influence Exerted by the Lacrimal Layer on Topographical Modeling System Records

Y. Iwabuchi,* H. Yamaguchi,* H. Shioya,* M. Kajita,* K. Kato,* and H. Takahashi† *Department of Ophthalmology, Fukushima Medical College, Japan, and †Esta Eye Clinic.

It has become possible to observe and record minor changes of the cornea owing to recent developments in the apparatus for measuring corneal shape, such as the topographical modeling system (TMS). However, we have some doubts about the reproducibility of the results of this system, especially with regard to the influence of the lacrimal layer (tear film). We set out to address the relationship between corneal shape and breakup time of tear film (BUT).

Autorefractometry, keratometry, corneal topography by TMS, and BUT were reexamined on selected subjects on different days but at similar time intervals. Examination was made immediately and 20, 40, and 60 seconds after nictitation, and without touching the subject's eyelid.

In the subjects with a BUT of more than 20 seconds, scarcely any change over time was observed in the values measured by autorefractometer and keratometer, but with-the-rule astigmatism in 1-D level was found, by TMS, to have developed after 20 to 40 seconds. Furthermore, there was a tendency for the symptom to recur immediately after nictitation as more time elapsed. These changes occurred earlier in the cases with a BUT as short as approximately 5 seconds.

We concluded that, even in the patient with a sufficiently long BUT, tear film seems to influence the findings obtained with high-precision measuring systems such as TMS. This influence is still more remarkable in the patient with insufficient tear film. To interpret TMS findings accurately, the practitioner must consider whether the cornea and tear film are being recorded in a constant state.

Influence of Contact Lens on Anterior Chamber Flare

H. Yamaguchi, Y. Iwabuchi, K. Kobari, H. Shioya, M. Kajita, and K. Kato Department of Ophthalmology, Fukushima Medical College, Japan

It is well-known that various influences are exerted on the cornea by a contact lens. The corneal endothelium exhibits a decreased average cellular area, increased variation coefficient, and decreased emerging rate of hexagonal cells. These changes may be attributable to decreased partial pressure of oxygen on the corneal surface, mechanical stimulation associated with attachment and removal of the contact lens, and nictitation.

We hypothesized that some change occurs in the anterior chamber by attachment of a contact lens, thus exerting an influence on corneal endothelial cells. To test this theory, we made assessments of the flare value of the anterior chamber.

Measurement of the flare of the anterior chamber was made with a laser flare cell meter (Kowa). Two subject groups were selected, one of which included 40 myopic eyes without ophthalmic disease (average age, 28.1 years) and the other 20 eyes with keratoconus (average age, 31.1 years).

The average flare values of the anterior chamber were 5.69 ± 1.22 (photon count/msec) in the myopic group and 6.73 ± 3.72 (photon count/msec) in the keratoconus group, both being within the range of normal values. No significant difference in the means of the values was obtained between the two groups.

From the fact that no change occurred in the flare value of the anterior chamber on attachment of a contact lens, we concluded that the conditional change in the anterior chamber may not influence the change in the corneal endothelium that occurs with attachment of a contact lens.

Children's Frequent Blinking and Dry Eye
Hao-Yung Yang,* Makoto Inoue,† Yukiko Yagi,‡ Ikuko Toda,‡ and Kazuo Tsubota‡ *Department of Ophthalmology, Keio University, Tokyo; †Department of Ophthalmology, Hino-Shiritsu Hospital; and ‡Department of Ophthalmology, Tokyo Dental College, Chiba, Japan

Children's frequent blinking is seen sometimes and has been considered a manifestation of underlying psychological conflict, reflex against light, a habit spasm, and a facial tic. We suggest that some of these cases are exacerbated by dry eye. We reviewed the records of 18 dry-eye patients younger than 15 years. Of these patients, we found 6 children (33 percent) exhibited frequent blinking. In these cases, tear film breakup time (BUT) was shortened, and there was an allergic conjunctivitis or mild form of vernal conjunctivitis present. Prescription of artificial tear eye drops and antiallergic medication relieved the frequent blinking in all cases. Based on these results, we believe dry eye must be included in the differential diagnosis of frequent blinking in a child.

■ Surgery and Complications

Suppression of Corneal Allograft Rejection: A Comparison of Cyclosporin and FK-506 Eye Drops
Astushi Kanai and Shuichi Akiyama   Department of Ophthalmology, Juntendo University School of Medicine, Tokyo, Japan

We conducted a comparative study of the effects of 0.05% cyclosporin (CYA) eye drops and 0.1% FK-506 eye drops in prolonging graft survival in a rabbit model of corneal graft rejection. The concentration of CYA in the cornea reached 1,300 ng/g at 24 hours, whereas the concentration of FK-506 in the cornea reached 370 ng/g 30 minutes after application, and 130 ng/g was present at 24 hours.

Thirty animals received corneal allografts, and skin grafts were also exchanged between pairs 14 days after the keratoplasty. We divided the subjects into three groups consisting of 10 eyes each. Group 1 was given 0.05% CYA, group 2 received 0.1% FK-506, and group 3 was given vehicle of CYA (alpha-cyclodextrin, 80 mg/ml) as a control. The drugs were applied four times daily over 50 days, and subjects were observed for an additional 50 days without any medication. Fifty days postoperatively, 2 of 10 eyes in the CYA group, 1 of 10 eyes in the FK-506 group, and 8 eyes in the control group exhibited graft rejection. After stopping the treatment, 2 eyes in the CYA group and 8 eyes in the FK-506 group experienced graft rejection.

Excimer Laser Partial External Trabeculectomy
Reiko Takeuchi, Masanobu Tanaka, Takayuki Takagi, and Yasuaki Kuwayama Department of Ophthalmology, Osaka University Medical School, Osaka, Japan

Partial external trabeculectomy (PET) using a 193-nm excimer laser has been proposed as a modified surgical filtration procedure. The excimer laser ablates the sclera, Schlemm's canal, and the outer portion of the trabecular meshwork, where the majority of aqueous outflow resistance is believed to occur. The flow of aqueous humor resulting when this resistance is eliminated prevents further ablation, leaves the rest of the trabecular meshwork unaffected, and results in nonpenetrating filtration.

Sixteen eyes with medically uncontrolled chronic open-angle glaucoma underwent PET, with follow-up from 6 to 19 months (10.5 ± 4.1 months). The mean preoperative intraocular pressure (IOP) was 27.9 ± 10.6 mm Hg. Postoperatively, 13 eyes (81 percent) had final IOPs of less than 21 mm Hg (mean, 15.8 ± 3.8 mm Hg); each had a cystic bleb. One eye required a subsequent conventional filtering procedure, and 2 eyes required Nd-YAG laser goniopuncture to control IOP. Gonioscopical examination visualized no anterior chamber penetration in any case. No unexpected complications were seen.

PET with a 193-nm excimer laser, used as a nonpenetrating filtering procedure, might reduce postoperative complications associated with a flat anterior chamber and inflammation. In addition, lack of thermal effect might be beneficial to the long-term maintenance of a filtering bleb. This procedure shows promise as a reasonable alternative to the present surgical management of glaucoma.

Harmonic Wave of YAG Laser for Keratectomy
Kazunori Miyata,[*] Akira Kakimoto,[*] Akihiro Horii,[†] and Yasuhiro Osakabe[‡] [*]Department of Ophthalmology and [†]Department of Precision Machinery Engineering, University of Tokyo School of Medicine, and [‡]Department of Pathology, Tokyo Medical College, Tokyo, Japan

Harmonic-wave YAG laser for keratectomy has been developed. The system consists of a Q-switched YAG laser and two nonlinear optical crystals. The first crystal converts the YAG laser beam (1,064 nm) into a beam with one-half the wavelength (532 nm), and the second crystal converts it into one-fourth the wavelength (266 nm).

The maximum converting efficiency of the second-harmonic YAG laser (532 nm) is 28 percent and that of the fourth harmonic YAG laser (266 nm) is 4.5 percent. The relationship between irradiation energy fluence and incision depth is linear at low energy. The relationship between the average number of irradiation pulses and incision depth is linear at 6 J/cm^2. Minimal thermal damage of the corneal tissue was observed with this fourth-harmonic YAG laser, similar to results with an excimer laser using KrF.

Thus, we concluded that this harmonic-wave YAG laser is as useful in laser corneal surgery as is excimer laser.

Surgical Correction of Congenital Ptosis
Ray S. Dixon and Edward R. O'Malley Grosse Pointe Ophthalmology, Grosse Pointe Park, Michigan

The surgical correction of congenital blepharoptosis is challenging because of the condition's possible variables, which include severity, symmetry, and the presence of associated phenomena. The ideal procedure should improve eyelid position and cosmesis without jeopardizing the cornea. Bilateral and equal surgical intervention gives the best outcome. Unilateral cases with good levator excursion are well-corrected by levator aponeurosis reinsertion, whereas those with poor excursion require bilateral mechanical repair. When levator excursion is fair, maximal levator surgery to include Whitnall's ligament is appropriate. The authors employ these guidelines. In addition, we have found that for suspension procedures, two triangular slings placed in the suborbicular plane, with precise placement of the exit and entry points, consistently result in a good functional and cosmetic outcome.

Orbital Rim Fractures
Ray S. Dixon Grosse Pointe Ophthalmology, Grosse Pointe Park, Michigan

The rim of the orbit is important for eyelid support, for maintaining position of the contents of the orbit (especially the globe), and for cosmesis. Its fracture, at times overshadowed by other bony trauma and swelling, requires specific clinical and radiological evaluations for detection. There are sequelae that are direct consequences of rim displacement. Repair may be indicated for functional or cosmetic reasons. When wall fracture is an extension from the rim, the rim instability and position may dictate the corrective surgical approach. In these cases, bone graft should be considered.

Corneal Transplantation for Perforating Corneal Diseases
Tadahiko Tsuru* and Mitsuru Sawa† *Department of Ophthalmology, University of Tokyo School of Medicine, and †Department of Ophthalmology, Nihon University School of Medicine, Tokyo, Japan

Nontraumatic corneal perforation is often intractable because of the underlying pathological conditions, such as collagen diseases, severe infection, and alkali burn. In many cases, the perforation is accompanied by iris prolapses, complicated cataracts, or vitreous herniations, and reconstructive keratoplasty is necessary to manage it.

We performed corneal transplantations to treat corneal perforations in 21 eyes of 16 patients. The causes of the perforations were corneal ulcers in 7 eyes, herpetic keratitis in 6 eyes, rheumatoid arthritis in 5 eyes, alkali burns in 2 eyes, and neurotrophic corneal ulcer in 1 eye. We performed penetrating keratoplasties in 16 eyes and lamellar keratoplasties in 5 eyes. Anterior vitrectomies and intracapsular cataract extractions were also done in 6 eyes and 2 eyes, respectively. All the perforated lesions were cured by the corneal transplantations, but only 4 eyes retained visual acuity equal to or better than 20/200.

Excimer Laser Superficial Keratectomy: Results of 1-Year Follow-Up
Keizo Takahashi,* Yuichi Ohashi,* and Shigeru Kinoshita† *Department of Ophthalmology, Osaka University Medical School, Osaka, and †Department of Ophthalmology, Kyoto Prefectural University of Medicine, Kyoto, Japan

The 193-nm excimer laser comprises a new modality for treating superficial corneal disorders. Using Exci-Med UV200LA (Summit Technology, 180 mJ/cm^2, 10 Hz), we performed 57 excimer laser superficial keratectomies in 48 patients with various corneal dystrophies or central opacities in the superficial stroma. The number of applied pulses ranged from 204 to 1,100, with optical zone diameter of 3.5 to 4.5 mm. Viscoelastic materials were used in case of surface smoothing. All patients achieved better or equal best-corrected visual acuity during the follow-up period of 1 year. The early postoperative course was uneventful. Late postoperative complications included a significant amount of hyperopic shifts, which occurred in all treated eyes and subepithelial scarring, which developed in only 1 eye. Corneal lesions recurred in 2 eyes.

Quantitative Evaluation of Postoperative Inflammation in Penetrating Keratoplasty
Mitsuru Sawa* and Kenji Urata† *Department of Ophthalmology, Nihon University School of Medicine, Tokyo, and †Department of Ophthalmology, Tokyo University School of Medicine, Tokyo, Japan

Aqueous protein concentration in eyes undergoing penetrating keratoplasty was determined using the laser flare cell meter. The subjects were divided into four groups, according to their disease: keratoconus, leukoma due to herpes or parenchymatous keratitis, bullous keratopathy, and corneal degeneration. Most eyes underwent keratoplasty alone, but several underwent keratoplasty with cataract extraction. Aqueous protein concentration increased in the early postoperative period, but it did not exceed more than 700 mg/dl, and it decreased over time. The keratoconus group had a lower protein concentration than other groups. The breakdown of the blood-aqueous barrier was not as severe with keratoplasty alone as opposed to keratoplasty and cataract extraction.

Long-Term Follow-Up Study of Cases Undergoing Anterior and Posterior Radial Keratotomy (Sato's Refractive Surgery)
Mitsuru Sawa,* Chikako Kimura,† Tsutomu Sato,‡ and Teruo Tanishima§ *Department of Ophthalmology, Nihon University School of Medicine, and Tokyo University School of Medicine, Tokyo; †Department of Ophthalmology, Toshiba Central Hospital, Tokyo; ‡Sato Eye Hospital, Yokohama; and §Hibiya Eye Clinic, Tokyo, Japan

Twenty-nine eyes undergoing anterior and posterior radial keratotomy for refractive correction were followed. Bullous keratopathy developed in 21 of 29 eyes over a period of 29 to 39 postoperative years. Endothelial cell density in 5 clear corneas averaged approximately 1,100 cells/mm^2 after more than 23 postoperative years. Twelve of 21 eyes with bullous keratopathy underwent penetrating keratoplasty, and 7 eyes developed graft failure within 7 years of this procedure.

Modified Method for Grafting in Keratoepithelioplasty
Mitsuru Sawa Department of Ophthalmology, Nihon University School of Medicine, Tokyo, Japan

A ring-shaped corneal tissue was obtained from a donor eye using a whole eye chamber. Internal incision was made using a 7- or 7.5-mm trephine, and the outer margin at the limbus was cut using a microblade. The excised corneal graft was cut into two halves, and each cut tissue was sutured at the limbal sclera of a recipient. At least two lenticles were taken from the inner area of the trephined incision of the donor and were sutured to cover the shortage of the ring graft. This modified method for grafting permitted covering the entire limbus in keratoepithelioplasty.

Histopathological Study of Corneoscleral Wounds in Self-Sealing Sutureless Cataract Extraction
Toshiro Shigemitsu and Yoshinao Majima Department of Ophthalmology, School of Medicine, Fujita Health University, Toyoake City, Japan

A morphological analysis was performed by means of scanning electron microscopy and light microscopy in rabbit eyes after they had undergone sutureless cataract extraction. Two types of sutureless cataract extraction were carried out in white rabbits. In one operation, an incision 5 mm long was made 0.5 mm from the corneal limbus, and entry into the anterior chamber was obtained at 1.5 mm to the clear cornea. In the other operation, an incision 5 mm long was made 2.5 mm from the limbus, and entry into the anterior chamber was obtained 0.5 mm to the clear cornea.

Eyeballs were removed 1, 3, 7, 14, 21, and 28 days after operation, and were examined. Inflammatory cell infiltration was notable until 2 weeks after either operation but was negligible after 4 weeks. Loss of corneal endothelial cells was observed at the wound until 14 days after either operation, but the corneal endothelium was repaired after 28 days. Aggregation of mesenchymal cells was clearly observed in the corneal and scleral stroma along the wound 14 days after either operation, but it too was absent after 28 days. The opening of the wound on the surface of the sclera was smaller after incision near the cornea than after incision near the sclera, but a small opening was observed in either case after 28 days. The wound generally showed tight union 3 days after either procedure except in the superficial layer of the sclera. The wound surface became obscure more than 14 days after either operation, and union of the wound was tighter still.

Index

Aberrant class II histocompatibility antigen expression, 4–6
Abstracts of the Pacific Ophthalmic Forum, 151–166
Acid, hyaluronic, 119–120
Acinar cell
  mimicking by, 7–12
  secretion and, 1
Acquired immunodeficiency syndrome, 3–4, 140–141
Adhesion molecules, cell, 137–138
Adhesive, tissue, 147–148
AIDS, 3–4, 140–141
Aldose reductase inhibitor, 122
Allergic conjunctivitis, 129–130
  keratoconjunctivitis sicca and, 38
Allergic keratoconjunctivitis, 54
Androgen, lacrimal gland influenced by, 20–23
Anesthesia, dry-eye and, 84–85
Anesthetic, dye staining and, 65
Anethole-trithione, 98
Antibiotic, Sjögren's syndrome and, 85
Antibody, Sjögren's syndrome and, 75
Anticholinergic side effects of drugs, 81
Antidepressant, side effects of, 81
Antifungal agent, 98
Antigen
  aberrant class II histocompatibility, 4–6
  human leukocyte, 83, 95–96
  Sjögren's syndrome and, 75, 83
Antihypertensive agents, 81
Antiinflammatory agent, 107
Antinuclear antibody, 75
Aqueous abnormality, 131–132
Argon laser, 146–147
Arthritis, rheumatoid, 76–77, 84
Artificial tears, 102–105
  new, 118–121
Autoantibody, 82–83
Autoimmunity
  of lacrimal gland, 1–18
    acinar cells and, 7–12

  chronic inflammation and, 1–3
  class II molecules and, 6–7
  histocompatibility antigen and, 4–6
  secretion and, 1
  T-cell activation and, 6
  viral infection and, 3–4
  Sjögren's syndrome and, 75–76

B lymphocyte
  malignant transformation and, 97
  Sjögren's syndrome and, 137
Bandage soft contact lenses, 107–109
Base abnormality, 132
Benzalkonium chloride, 104
Bicarbonate, in tear film, 30–35
Biliary cirrhosis, 79
Bion Tear, 103
Biopsy, salivary gland, 94–95
Blepharitis
  contact lenses and, 129–130
  indications of, 44
  keratoconjunctivitis sicca versus, 38, 53
  mimicking dry eye, 82
Blepharoplasty, 110–111
Blepharospasm, 82
Blink rate, 116–117
Blinking
  contact lenses and, 133
  dry eye and, 82
Bromhexine, 98
Bulbar conjunctiva, examination of, 44

Calcium, in tear film, 30–33
Candidiasis, treatment of, 98
Carbachol, 8
Cathepsin B, 9–10
Cathepsin D, 9–10
Cell
  acinar
    mimicking by, 7–12
    secretion and, 1
  dye staining and, 60, 65
  goblet, 62
  lymphoblastoid, 5

Sjögren's syndrome and, 83, 137–143
T. *See* T lymphocyte
Cell adhesion molecules, 137–138
Chemosensory function alterations, 93
Chlorhexidine, 104
Chloride ions
  in saliva, 93
  in tears, 20
Chlorobutanol, 104
Cicatricial pemphigoid, 54–55
Cirrhosis, 79
Class II molecules, antigen processing of, 6–7
Collagen punctal plug
  keratoconjunctivitis sicca and, 41
  types of, 148
Conjunctival examination, 44
Conjunctivitis. *See also* Keratoconjunctivitis sicca
  allergic, 129–130
  ocular surface disease and, 54
Contact lenses, 129–136
  bandage, 107–109
Copenhagen criteria for Sjögren's syndrome, 75
Copolymer punctal plug, 149–150
Cornea
  examination of, 44–45
  ocular surface disease and, 54
  preservatives affecting, 104
Corneal prosthesis, 110
Cotton thread test, 46
CREST, 79
Cyanoacrylate tissue adhesive, 147–148
Cyclosporine A, 124
Cytokine, 137–138

Dermatochalasis, 43
  keratoconjunctivitis sicca versus, 38
Dermatomyositis, 79
Diethylstilbestrol, 21–22
Dihydrotestosterone, 20, 23
Drug-induced dry-eye symptoms, 41–42, 81
Dry eye. *See also* Keratoconjunctivitis sicca; Sjögren's syndrome
  contact lenses and, 129–134
  definition of, 101–102
  drug therapy causing, 41–42, 81
  systemic disease associated with, 71–87. *See also* Systemic disease associated with dry eye
  treatment of, 102–113

antiinflammatory agents for, 107
artificial tears for, 102–105, 118–121
  choice of, 111
  corneal epithelium and, 122–124
  estrogens for, 110
  hydrophilic lenses for, 107–109
  immunotherapy for, 124
  lubricants for, 105
  moisture glasses and, 117–118
  surface, 109
  surgery in, 110–111
  tear preservation in, 105–107
  tear stimulation in, 105
  tear viscosity and, 109–110
Dry mouth, 89–100. *See also* Sjögren's syndrome; Xerostomia
Duct, parotid, transplantation of, 110
Dye eye, keratoconjunctivitis sicca versus, 37
Dye staining of ocular surface, 60–66
Dysphagia, 93

Electrocautery, 145–146
Electrolytes
  salivary, 93
  in tear film, 27–36
Electrophoresis, of tear film, 49
Endophthalmitis, bandage lenses causing, 109
Enlargement of salivary gland, 91
Environmental factors in Sjögren's syndrome, 140–141
Epidermal growth factor, 122
Epithelium
  fluorescein staining of, 48
  rose bengal staining of, 60–66
  treatment for, 122–124
Epstein-Barr virus
  autoimmunity and, 3
  oral disease and, 95
  Sjögren's syndrome and, 140
Estrogen
  keratoconjunctivitis sicca and, 110
  Sjögren's syndrome and, 19–20
Evaporation of tear film, 49, 115–116
Exophthalmos, Graves' disease and, 43
Extended-wear contact lenses, 133
Eyelid, examination of, 43–44

Ferning of tear film, 48–49
Film, tear. *See* Tear film
Fluid therapy, Sjögren's syndrome and, 85

Fluorescein
  chemical structure of, 61
  tear breakup time and, 46
Fluorescent light, photophobia and, 51–52
Fluorophotometry, 46
Freeman punctal plug, 148

Gelatin implant, 147
Gland
  lacrimal. *See* Lacrimal gland
  meibomian
    abnormalities of, 102
    contact lenses and, 130
    examination of, 44
    lipid abnormality and, 131
    tear film osmolarity and, 27–36
  salivary
    dysfunction of, 90–93
    Sjögren's syndrome and, 43, 72–74, 83
Glasses, moisture, 117–118
Goblet cell, 62
Graft-versus-host disease, 82
Granzyme A, 141–142
Growth factor, epidermal, 122

Halide, 62
High-viscosity methylcellulose, 120–121
Histocompatibility antigen, aberrant class II, 4–6
Hormonal influences on lacrimal gland, 19–25
  androgens and, 20–23
  prolactin and, 22–23
Human immunodeficiency virus infection, 3–4, 140–141
Human leukocyte antigen
  aberrant class II, 4–6
  oral disease and, 95–96
  Sjögren's syndrome and, 83
Human T-cell lymphotropic virus-I, 140
Humidity, moisture glasses and, 117–118
Hyaluronic acid, 119–120
Hydrophilic contact lenses, 107–109

Iatrogenic disease, preservatives causing, 104
Immunoglobulin, 96
Immunology of salivary gland, 96–97
Immunotherapy, 124–125
Implant, intracanalicular, 147
Infection
  oral disease and, 95–96
  Sjögren's syndrome and, 80–81
  viral
    autoimmunity and, 3–4
    oral disease and, 95–96
    Sjögren's syndrome and, 140
Infiltrative disease, 79–80
  lymphocytic, 72–73, 82–84
Inflammation
  chronic, 1–3
  indications of, 44
  keratoconjunctivitis sicca and, 38
Insert, artificial tear, 103–104
Interferon alpha, 124–125, 141
Interferon gamma
  class II molecule expression and, 10
  Sjögren's syndrome and, 83
Intracanalicular gelatin implant, 147
Intracellular adhesion molecule, 137–139
Intracellular pools of plasma membrane constituents, 7–9
Invasive tear breakup time, 46
Irritant keratoconjunctivitis, 53–54

Jones's test, 45–46

Keratoconjunctivitis sicca, 38–56. *See also* Sjögren's syndrome
  allergic, 54
  antiinflammatory agents for, 107
  bandage contact lenses for, 107–109
  blepharitis and, 53
  causes of, 37–38
  clinical examination for, 43–45
  clinical tests for, 45–48
  decreasing of tear viscosity in, 109–110
  dye staining pattern in, 66
  estrogens in, 110
  laboratory tests for, 48–51
  lubricants for, 41, 105
  other syndromes versus, 51–54
  patient history of, 38–43
  preservatives causing, 104–105
  punctal plugs for, 41, 105–107
  Sjögren's syndrome and, 72–73
  tear film osmolarity and, 27–35
  tear secretion and, 102
  toxic or irritant, 53–54
  treatment trials for, 51
Kidney disease, 75

Labial salivary gland biopsy, 94–95
Lacrimal gland
  autoimmunity of, 1–18
  acinar cells and, 7–12

chronic inflammation and, 1–3
class II molecules and, 6–7
histocompatibility antigen and, 4–6
secretion and, 1
T-cell activation and, 6
viral infection and, 3–4
hormonal influences on, 19–25
size of, 44
tear film osmolarity and, 27–36
Lacrisert, 103–104
Lactoferrin, in tear film, 49
Laser cautery, 146–147
Lenses, contact, 129–136
bandage, 107–109
Leukocyte antigen, human, aberrant class II, 4–6
Light, photophobia and, 51–52
Lip, salivary gland biopsy of, 94–95
Lipid abnormality, 131
Lissamine green B, 62
chemical structure of, 61
Lubricant, 41, 105
Lupus erythematosus, systemic, 77–78
Lymphoblastoid cells, 5
Lymphocyte, T. *See* T lymphocyte
Lymphocytic infiltrate, 72–73, 82–84
Lymphoma, Sjögren's syndrome and, 97
Lymphoproliferation, 141
Lysozyme, in tear film, 49

MAChRs, 21–23
Magnesium, in tear film, 30, 32–33
Malignant transformation, 97
Meibomian gland
abnormalities of, 102
contact lenses and, 130
examination of, 44
lipid abnormality and, 131
tear film osmolarity and, 27–36
MEM. *See* Mucin-like glycoproteins
Membrane, plasma, intracellular pools of, 7–9
Methylcellulose, high-viscosity, 120–121
Mikulicz's disease, 43, 72
Moisture glasses, 117–118
Molecule, class II, 6–7
Motor function alterations, 93
Mouth
diseases of, 89–100. *See also* Oral disease
dryness of, 43
Mucin abnormality, 132
Mucin-like glycoproteins, 58–59, 62–63
Muscarinic, cholinergic receptors, 21, 23

Na^+,K^+-ATPase, androgens and, 21–22
Na,K-ATPase pump units, 7
Nephritis, Sjögren's syndrome and, 75
Noninvasive tear breakup time, 47
Nystatin, for candidiasis, 98

Occlusion, punctal, methods of, 145–150
Ocular surface
blinking and, 116–117, 133
disease of, treatment of, 101–111
diseases of, 54–55
dye staining of, 60–66
epithelium and, 57–59
histological evaluation of, 49–50
tear film and, 37, 57–59
Oral disease, 75, 89–100
causes of, 95–96
immunology of, 96–97
keratoconjunctivitis sicca and, 42–43
malignancy and, 97
salivary gland, 90–93
biopsy and, 94–95
sensory and motor function and, 93
treatment of, 97–98
Orbital vasculitis, 78
Osmolarity of tear film, 27–36, 48
contact lenses and, 133–134

Pacific Ophthalmic Forum, abstracts of, 151–166
Papilla, of tongue, 91–92
Parotid duct transplantation, 110
Pemphigoid, 54–55
Perforin, 141–142
Peritron, 46
pH, of tear film, 48
Phakic contact lenses, 133
Photophobia, 51–52
Photothrombosis, 61
Pilocarpine, 98
Plasma membrane, 7–9
Plug, punctal, 41, 105–107
collagen, 148
copolymer, 149–150
intracanalicular gelatin, 147
silicone, 148–149
Polymyositis, 79
Potassium, in tear film, 30–35
Potassium ions, 20
Preservative, corneal disease and, 104
Progressive systemic sclerosis, 79
Prolactin, 24
lacrimal gland influenced by, 20–23
Prosthesis, corneal, 110

Protein, in tear film, 49
Pseudolymphoma, 97
Pseudomonas aeruginosa, RDG peptide and, 120
Punctal occlusion, 41, 105–107
  methods of, 145–150

Radiation therapy, 82
Renal disease, 75
Respiratory system, 75
RGD peptide, 120
Rheumatoid arthritis, 76–77, 84
Rose bengal staining, 47–48, 60–66

Saliva, 92
Salivary gland
  dysfunction of, 90–93
  Sjögren's syndrome and, 43, 72–74, 83
San Diego criteria for Sjögren's syndrome, 74–75
San Francisco criteria for Sjögren's syndrome, 72–74
Sarcoidosis, 82
Schirmer's test, 45–46
  contact lenses and, 129
Sclerosis, progressive systemic, 79
Secretion, lacrimal, 1
Sensory function alterations, 93
Sexual dimorphism of Sjögren's syndrome, 19
Sialadenitis, 74–75
Sicca syndrome. *See* Keratoconjunctivitis sicca
Silicone punctal plug, 41, 148–149
Sjögren's syndrome
  background of, 71–72
  cellular activation in, 137–143
  cirrhosis and, 79
  classification of, 72–75
  dermatomyositis and, 79
  differential diagnosis of, 79–82
  extraglandular manifestations of, 75
  high-viscosity methylcellulose in, 121
  inflammation and, 1–2
  keratoconjunctivitis sicca and, 42–43
  oral symptoms of, 89–100
    causes of, 95–96
    malignancy and, 97
    salivary gland biopsy and, 94–95
    salivary gland dysfunction and, 90–93
    sensory and motor function and, 93
    treatment of, 97–98
  pathogenesis of, 82–84

progressive systemic sclerosis and, 79
rheumatoid arthritis and, 76–77
rose bengal staining and, 60–61
systemic lupus erythematosus with, 77–78
treatment of, 84–85
Slit-lamp examination, 44
Smell, sense of, 93
Sodium
  in saliva, 93
  in tear film, 30–34
Sodium hyaluronate solution, 103
Soft contact lenses
  bandage, 107–109
  osmolarity and, 133–134
Staining of ocular surface, 47–48, 60–66
Stenosis, 29
Steroid, 85
Stevens-Johnson syndrome, 54
Stimulant
  salivary, 98
  tear, 105
Sulforhodamine B, 61
Surface. *See* Ocular surface
Surgery for dry-eye syndromes, 110–111
Swallowing, difficulty with, 93
Systemic disease associated with dry eye, 71–87
  biliary cirrhosis as, 79
  dermatomyositis as, 79
  progressive systemic sclerosis as, 79
  rheumatoid arthritis as, 76–77
  Sjögren's syndrome as, 71–76
    differential diagnosis of, 79–82
    pathogenesis of, 82–84
    treatment of, 84–85
  systemic lupus erythematosus as, 77–78
Systemic lupus erythematosus, 77–78

T lymphocyte
  aberrant histocompatibility antigen expression and, 4–5
  accessory signals for, 6
  inflammation and, 1–3
  malignant transformation and, 97
  salivary gland and, 96
  Sjögren's syndrome and, 82–83, 137
Tarsal conjunctiva reaction, contact lenses and, 130
Tarsorrhaphy, 110–111
Taste, sense of, 93
Tear
  artificial, 102–105

new, 118–121
  decreased production of, 101–102
  measurement of, 45–46
  stability of, 46–47
  volume abnormality of, 131–132
Tear film
  chemical composition of, 49
  components of, 102
  contact lenses and, 133
  dry eye and, 37
  evaporation of, 49
  ferning of, 48–49
  integrity of, 47–48
  lipid abnormality and, 131
  osmolarity of, 27–36, 48
    contact lenses and, 133–134
  pH of, 48
  unstable, 60
Temperature, intracellular pools of plasma membrane constituents and, 8–9
Thimerosal, 104
Thyroid disorder, 43
Tissue adhesive, cyanoacrylate, 147–148
Tongue, Sjögren's syndrome and, 91–92
Topical lubricant, 41, 105

Toxic keratoconjunctivitis, 53–54
Transplantation, parotid duct, 110
Trichiasis, 44
Tumor necrosis factor, 139

Unstable tear film, 60

Vascular cell adhesion molecule, 137–139
Vasculitis, Sjögren's syndrome and, 78
Very late antigen antibodies, 139
Viral infection
  autoimmunity and, 3–4
  oral disease and, 95–96
  Sjögren's syndrome and, 140
Visco Tears, 120
Viscosity of tears, decreasing of, 109–110
Vital dye staining, 60–66
Vitamin A, 122, 124
VLA antibodies, 139

Xerostomia. *See also* Oral disease
  keratoconjunctivitis sicca and, 42–43
  salivary gland dysfunction and, 90–91
  Sjögren's syndrome and, 75

Future Issues

Volume 34, 1994

Spring (No. 2)

CATARACT SURGERY
Jack M. Dodick, M.D., Guest Editor

Summer (No. 3)

ADVANCES IN OPHTHALMIC DIAGNOSTIC TECHNOLOGY
Frederick A. Jakobiec, M.D., Guest Editor

Fall (No. 4)

REFRACTIVE SURGERY
Olivia Serdarevic, M.D., Guest Editor

U.S. Postal Service Statement of Ownership, Management and Circulation (required by 39 U.S.C. 3685). 1A. Title of publication: INTERNATIONAL OPHTHALMOLOGY CLINICS. 1B. Publication no.: 00208167. 2. Date of filing: October 1, 1993. 3. Frequency of issue: quarterly. 3A. No. of issues published annually: 4. 3B. Annual subscription price: $90.00. 4. Complete mailing address of known office of publication (street, city, county, state and ZIP code) (not printers): 34 Beacon Street, Boston, Suffolk County, Massachusetts 02108-1493. 5. Complete mailing address of the headquarters or general business offices of the publishers (not printers): 34 Beacon Street, Boston, Suffolk County, Massachusetts 02108-1493. 6. Full names and complete mailing address of publisher, editor, and managing editor (this item *must not* be blank): Publisher (name and complete mailing address): Little, Brown and Company, Inc., 34 Beacon Street, Boston, Massachusetts 02108-1493. Editor (name and complete mailing address): Gilbert Smolin, MD, and Mitchell Friedlaender, MD, 1001 Sneath Lane, Room 206, San Bruno, CA 94066. Managing Editor (name and complete mailing address): Maureen Hurley, Little, Brown and Company, 34 Beacon Street, Boston, Massachusetts 02108-1493. 7, 8. Owner (If owned by a corporation, its name and address must be stated and also immediately thereunder the names and addresses of stockholders owning or holding 1 percent or more of total amount of stock. If not owned by a corporation, the names and addresses of the individual owners must be given. If owned by a partnership or other unincorporated firm, its name and address, as well as that of each individual must be given. If the publication is published by a nonprofit organization, its name and address must be stated.) (Item must be completed): Full name: Little, Brown and Company (Incorporated). Complete mailing address: 34 Beacon Street, Boston, Massachusetts 02108-1493, which is a direct wholly-owned subsidiary of Time Inc., 1271 Avenue of the Americas, New York, NY 10020, which is a wholly-owned subsidiary of Time Warner Inc., 75 Rockefeller Plaza, New York, NY 10019. To the best of Time Warner's knowledge, the names and addresses of stockholders owning or holding 1 percent or more of the stock of Time Warner Inc. are as follows: Depository Trust Co., P.O. Box 20, Bowling Green Station, New York, NY (as of 8/25/93)*; Alliance Capital Management L.P., 1345 Avenue of the Americas, New York, NY*; The Capital Group, Inc., 333 South Hope Street, Los Angeles, CA*; Chancellor Capital Management, Inc., 153 East 53rd Street, New York, NY*; Eagle Asset Management, Inc., 880 Carillon Parkway, St. Petersburg, FL*; Fidelity Management & Research Co., 82 Devonshire Street, Boston, MA*; First Interstate Bank of California, 707 Wilshire Boulevard, Los Angeles, CA*; Henry Luce Foundation, Inc., 111 West 50th Street, New York, NY (as of 2/15/93); IDS Financial Services, Inc., IDS Tower 10, Minneapolis, MN*; Indiana National Bank Co., Trustee, P.O. Box 1832, Indianapolis, IN (as of 8/25/93)*; Investors Research Corp., 4500 Main Street, Kansas City, MO*; J.P. Morgan Investment Management (U.S.), 60 Wall Street, New York, NY*; Jencik & Co., c/o Morgan Guaranty Trust Co. of New York, Box 1479, Church Street Station, New York, NY (as of 8/25/93)*; Kray & Co., One Financial Place, 440 S. LaSalle Street, Chicago, IL (as of 8/25/93)*; Lynch & Mayer, Inc., 650 Fifth Avenue, New York, NY*; Neuberger & Berman Pension Management, Inc., 605 Third Avenue, New York, NY*; New York State Common Retirement Fund, A. E. Smith Building, South Swan Street, Albany, NY; Oppenheimer Capital, One World Trade Center, New York, NY*; Prudential Investment Advisors, Five Prudential Plaza, Newark, NJ*; RCM Capital Management, Four Embarcadero Center, San Francisco, CA*; The Seagram Company Ltd., 1430 Peel Street, Montreal, Quebec, CANADA (as of 5/26/93); SIOR & Co., c/o Bankers Trust Co., and Bankers Trust Company, Box 704, New York, NY (as of 8/25/93)*; TIAA-CREF Investment Management, Inc., 730 Third Avenue, New York, NY; Wells Fargo Nikko Investment Advisors, 45 Fremont Street, San Francisco, CA*. To the best of Time Warner's knowledge, as of August 31, 1993, both the Depository Trust Co., P.O. Box 20, Bowling Green Station, New York, NY*, and BHC Communications, Inc., 600 Madison Avenue, New York, NY, hold of record 1 percent or more of the debt securities of Time Warner Inc. *Believed to be held for the account of one or more security holders. 9. For completion by nonprofit organizations authorized to mail at special rates (Section 423.12, DMM only). The purpose, function, and nonprofit status of this organization and the exempt status for Federal income tax purposes (Check one): (1) Has not changed during preceding 12 months; (2) Has changed during preceding 12 months (If changed, publisher must submit explanation of change with this statement.): None. 10. Extent and nature of circulation: A. Total no. copies (net press run): average no. copies each issue during preceding 12 months, 2471; actual no. copies of single issue published nearest to filing date, 2429. B. Paid circulation: 1. Sales through dealers and carriers, street vendors and counter sales: average no. copies each issue during preceding 12 months, 42; actual no. copies of single issue published nearest to filing date, 53. 2. Mail subscription: average no. copies each issue during preceding 12 months, 1595; actual no. copies of single issue published nearest to filing date, 1656. C. Total paid circulation (sum of 10B1 and 10B2): average no. copies each issue during preceding 12 months, 1637; actual no. copies of single issue published nearest to filing date, 1709. D. Free distribution by mail, carrier or other means, samples, complimentary, and other free copies: average no. copies each issue during preceding 12 months, 111; actual no. copies of single issue published nearest to filing date, 90. E. Total distribution (sum of C and D): average no. copies each issue during preceding 12 months, 1748; actual no. copies of single issue published nearest to filing date, 1799. F. Copies not distributed: 1. Office use, left over, unaccounted, spoiled after printing: average no. copies each issue during preceding 12 months, 723; actual no. copies of single issue published nearest to filing date, 630. 2. Return from news agents: average no. copies each issue during preceding 12 months, none; actual no. copies of single issue published nearest to filing date, none. G. Total (sum of E, F1 and 2—should equal net press run shown in A): average no. copies each issue during preceding 12 months, 2471; actual no. copies of single issue published nearest to filing date, 2429. H. I certify that the statements made by me above are correct and complete. Signature and title of editor, publisher, business manager, or owner: Christine Finn, Business Manager.